ENDOCRINOLOGY RESEARCH AND CLINICAL DEVELOPMENTS

DIABETIC FOOT

PREVENTION AND TREATMENT

ENDOCRINOLOGY RESEARCH AND CLINICAL DEVELOPMENTS

Additional books and e-books in this series can be found on Nova's website under the Series tab.

ENDOCRINOLOGY RESEARCH AND CLINICAL DEVELOPMENTS

DIABETIC FOOT

PREVENTION AND TREATMENT

GIANNI ROMANO
EDITOR

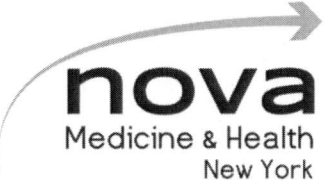

Copyright © 2019 by Nova Science Publishers, Inc.

All rights reserved. No part of this book may be reproduced, stored in a retrieval system or transmitted in any form or by any means: electronic, electrostatic, magnetic, tape, mechanical photocopying, recording or otherwise without the written permission of the Publisher.

We have partnered with Copyright Clearance Center to make it easy for you to obtain permissions to reuse content from this publication. Simply navigate to this **publication's** page on Nova's website and locate the "Get Permission" button below the title description. This button is linked directly to the title's permission page on copyright.com. Alternatively, you can visit copyright.com and search by title, ISBN, or ISSN.

For further questions about using the service on copyright.com, please contact:
Copyright Clearance Center
Phone: +1-(978) 750-8400   Fax: +1-(978) 750-4470   E-mail: info@copyright.com

NOTICE TO THE READER

The Publisher has taken reasonable care in the preparation of this book, but makes no expressed or implied warranty of any kind and assumes no responsibility for any errors or omissions. No liability is assumed for incidental or consequential damages in connection with or arising out of information contained in this book. The Publisher shall not be liable for any special, consequential, or exemplary damages resulting, in whole or in part, from the **readers'** use of, or reliance upon, this material. Any parts of this book based on government reports are so indicated and copyright is claimed for those parts to the extent applicable to compilations of such works.

Independent verification should be sought for any data, advice or recommendations contained in this book. In addition, no responsibility is assumed by the Publisher for any injury and/or damage to persons or property arising from any methods, products, instructions, ideas or otherwise contained in this publication.

This publication is designed to provide accurate and authoritative information with regard to the subject matter covered herein. It is sold with the clear understanding that the Publisher is not engaged in rendering legal or any other professional services. If legal or any other expert assistance is required, the services of a competent person should be sought. FROM A DECLARATION OF PARTICIPANTS JOINTLY ADOPTED BY A COMMITTEE OF THE AMERICAN BAR ASSOCIATION AND A COMMITTEE OF PUBLISHERS.

Additional color graphics may be available in the e-book version of this book.

Library of Congress Cataloging-in-Publication Data

ISBN: 978-1-53616-266-0

Published by Nova Science Publishers, Inc. † New York

Contents

Preface		**vii**
Chapter 1	Machine Vision for Early Diabetes Diagnosis *Punal M Arabi and Gayatri Joshi*	**1**
Chapter 2	Clinical Applications of Mesenchymal Stem Cells in Non-Healing Diabetic Foot Ulcers (DFUs): An Effective Treatment *Surjya Narayan Dash, Nihar Ranjan Dash and Prakash Chandra Mohapatra*	**19**
Chapter 3	Are Antimicrobial Peptides the Answer for Diabetic Foot Infection Management? *Raquel Santos, Luís Tavares and Manuela Oliveira*	**51**
Chapter 4	Prospective on Advanced DFU Therapies: Identifying Alternatives to Conventional Therapy Based on Current Research *Isa Serrano, Raquel Santos, Rui Soares, Luis Tavares and Manuela Oliveira*	**81**

Chapter 5	The Effects of Social Support and Hope in the Healing of Diabetic Foot Ulcers Treated with Standard Care *Ayfer Peker Karatoprak and Süreyya Karaöz*	**151**
Index		**171**
Related Nova Publications		**175**

PREFACE

Diabetic Foot: Prevention and Treatment first proposes a noninvasive screening method for diabetes based on the thermoregulation of the peroneal vessel. Since diabetes affects the proneal vessel of the patients significantly, the thermoregulatory behavior of peroneal vessel is studied for induced hot and cold stress in this work.

Next, the authors highlight recent findings in the area of human mesenchymal stem cells sources, their differentiation ability, immunogenicity, adaptation to the microenvironment, as well as use in human clinical trials.

The authors also propose that, given the increasing prevalence of antibiotic resistant pathogens and the failure of antibiotic-exclusive therapeutics in the treatment of diabetic foot infections, combinations of antimicrobial peptides and antibiotics may be a potential treatment alternative.

Advanced diabetic foot ulcer therapies are explored based on current research. Recent studies show that diabetic patients have a 25% risk of developing diabetic foot ulcers in their lifetime.

Lastly, a study was carried out to investigate the effects of social support on the reduction of wound size after four weeks of treatment with standard care in patients with Grade B, Stage I diabetic foot ulcer.

Chapter 1 - Diabetic mellitus is a disorder of metabolism which is characterized by the elevated sugar levels in the blood over a prolonged period. There are three major types of diabetes namely type I, type II and gestational diabetes. According to senses taken in 2017, 8.8% of adult population worldwide was estimated to be diabetic which would shoot up to 9.9% by 2045, i.e about 6042 million of people would be affected worldwide. If diabetes is left untreated, it may lead to various diseases like kidney stone, diabetic retinopathy, diabetic neuropathy, stroke and heart attack. The people with diabetic neuropathy gradually lose sensitivity of the nervous system all over the body. Peripheral neuropathy is the most common type of diabetic neuropathy which is characterized by the loss of sensitivity in arms, hands, legs, feet and toes. If neuropathy in the foot is left untreated, it would increase the chances of occurrence of foot ulcers, infection and amputation of the limb. To save the patients from these complications and to ensure the quality of the life of them, there is a need for early diagnosis. This research work aims at proposing a non-invasive screening method for diabetes which is based on the thermoregulation of the peroneal vessel. Since diabetes affects the proneal vessel of the patients significantly, in this work the thermoregulatory behavior of peroneal vessel is studied for induced hot and cold stress. The study involved 20 subjects, out of which five persons are healthy or non-diabetic persons and the remaining 15 persons are of three categories namely patients with diabetes for less than 10 years, patients with diabetes for greater than 10 years, and patients with neuropathy; each category has five persons participating in this study. The results obtained show the feasibility of disease screening by the proposed method although it is to be improved for further classification of the stages of disease progression and accuracy. From the results, it is seen that the thermoregulatory response of the peroneal blood vessel in the leg to the cold stress is more meaningful as a disease marker compared to hot stress. The accuracy of the proposed method is found be 75% for cold stress for a response time window of 2 minutes.

Chapter 2 - Diabetes Mellitus is the condition where the level of sugar in blood is high. There are many complications of diabetes, Diabetic Foot Ulcer (DFU) being one of the most common complications of long-standing diabetes. Majority of the patients with diabetes foot ulcer (DFU) advance to amputations. DFU has emerged as one of the leading causes of mortality and morbidity and has a great financial implication on individual and the society. Therapeutic application of autologous BM-derived Mesenchymal stem cells (MSCs) have revolutionized the field of regenerative medicine and emerged as a promising therapeutic strategy to treat DFU. MSCs have multi-lineage differentiation potential and upon implantation they secrete cytokines that promote cell recruitment, immunomodulation, extracellular matrix remodeling, angiogenesis, and neuroregeneration facilitating wound healing. However, more detailed clinical studies and post-implantation follow up is required before it is used as cell replacement therapy (CRT) for nonhealing ulcers of the lower extremities in a larger context. This chapter highlights recent findings in the areas of hMSCs (human MSCs) sources, its differentiation ability, immunogenicity, adaptation to the microenvironment by secreting paracrine factors and its use in human clinical trials in DFUs.

Chapter 3 - Diabetes *mellitus* is a serious health problem that has shown an increasing prevalence in the last decades, affecting more than 422 million people globally nowadays. As a consequence of multiple pathophysiological factors, namely neuropathy, vasculopathy and immunopathy, the lifetime risk for diabetic patients of developing a foot ulcer can be as high as 25%. Approximately half of these ulcers can become clinically infected, usually by opportunistic pathogens, including both aerobic and anaerobic bacteria and yeasts. Due to local microenvironmental conditions unfavorable to wound healing, infected ulcers may result in purulent discharge, intense inflammation and progressive tissue damage. Several bacteria are related with diabetic foot infections (DFIs), mainly *Staphylococcus* spp., *Enterococcus* spp., *Streptococcus* spp., *Enterobacteriaceae*, *Pseudomonas* spp., *Acinetobacter* spp. and *Peptoniphilus* spp. These species have the ability to express numerous virulence factors that are putatively involved in their pathogenicity, including quorum-sensing molecules and biofilm structures. Moreover, DFI pathogens are known for their antibiotic resistance profile. The increasing prevalence of multidrug resistant isolates, formation of biofilms and inadequate wound healing found in DFIs may impair the successful outcome of conventional anti-infectious therapeutics in these patients. In fact, foot gangrene subsequent to a non-healing DFI is nowadays the leading cause of non-traumatic lower limb amputations. Antimicrobial peptides (AMPs) have emerged as a potential strategy to be used in combination with or as an alternative to conventional antibiotherapy in the management of chronic DFIs. AMPs are amphipathic molecules containing cationic and hydrophobic amino acid residues, enabling them to form non-specific interactions with the negatively charged bacterial membranes. There are several studies available regarding the activity of these small peptides, providing information on their antimicrobial spectrum, mechanisms of action and biological effects in wound healing. Nisin and pexiganan are two of the most promising AMPs for application against antibiotic resistant bacteria. Both nisin and pexiganan are able to disrupt prokaryotic membranes, inducing a fast killing of bacteria. Nisin binds to the peptidoglycan precursor lipid II, inhibiting cell wall synthesis and promoting pore formation on bacterial cytoplasmic membranes; on the other hand, pexiganan exerts its antibacterial effect via toroidal pore formation. The multiple mechanisms of action, the quick onset of activity and the low specificity in terms of molecular targets decreases the tendency of bacteria to develop resistance towards AMPs. Given the increasing prevalence of antibiotic resistant pathogens and, consequently, the failure of antibiotic-exclusive therapeutics in DFIs treatment, combinations involving AMPs and antibiotics may be a potential treatment alternative in a near future.

Chapter 4 - Diabetes *mellitus* (DM) is one of the most epidemic chronic diseases worldwide. From 1980 to 2014, there was a global increase of the disease prevalence, reaching 314 million adults aged over 18 years, a number which is expected to double by the year 2030. Recent studies show that diabetic patients have a 25% risk of developing diabetic foot ulcers (DFU) in their lifetime. Most (40-80%) DFU become infected, usually by polymicrobial populations, delaying wound healing and contributing to their chronicity. In 15% to 27% of the cases, DFU development leads to minor or major amputations of lower limbs, which in half of the cases are due to infection. As these amputations are a major cause of morbidity and mortality, new strategies to promote wound healing are urgent. Several advanced DFU therapies are being developed and include novel antiseptics, bio-engineered skin, negative pressure wound therapy, electrical stimulation, recombinant human platelet-derived growth factor, hyperbaric oxygen therapy, granulocyte-colony stimulating factor, low-level light therapy, and bacteriophage therapy. From these, only bio-engineered skin and negative pressure are recommended for DFU treatment. This review will discuss advanced DFU therapies based on current research.

Chapter 5 - *Aim: This study was carried out to investigate* the effects of "Social Support" and "Hope" on 50% reduction of wound size after four weeks of treatment with standard care in patients with Grade B, Stage I diabetic foot ulcer. *Methods:* The study population was composed of patients with Grade B, Stage I diabetic foot ulcers. The *study sample included 34 patients*, aged ≥40 years, with type 2 diabetes, HbA1c concentration of >7%. This *study used four data collection tools including* two *questionnaire and Beck Hopelessness Scale (BHS); Multidimensional Scale of Perceived Social Support (MSPSS).* All *patients received evidence-based standard* care. W*ound surface area was measured at days* 1 and 30 to determine whether 50% percent decrease has been achieved. T *test, correlation analysis, and chi-square test were used for data analysis. Findings: A positive correlation was found between* family social support and healing percentage ($r = 406$, $p = 0.01$). A*ccording to BHS,* patients with wounds healed over 50% in size had mild, and those with wounds healed less than 50% had moderate scores. There was a *negative correlation between social support and hopelessness* ($r = -449$, $p = 0.01$). A *negative correlation was found with social support from the family* ($r = -539$, $p = 0.01$) and *the friends* ($r = -457$, $p = 0.01$), and hopelessness. *Conclusion:* Social support and high motivation had a positive effect on wound healing in patients with diabetic foot ulcers. Family social support *affects healing in a positive way, but hopelessness in a negative way.*

In: Diabetic Foot: Prevention and Treatment ISBN: 978-1-53616-266-0
Editor: Gianni Romano © 2019 Nova Science Publishers, Inc.

Chapter 1

MACHINE VISION FOR EARLY DIABETES DIAGNOSIS

Punal M Arabi and Gayatri Joshi*
Department of BME, ACS College of Engineering,
Bangalore, Karnataka

ABSTRACT

Diabetic mellitus is a disorder of metabolism which is characterized by the elevated sugar levels in the blood over a prolonged period. There are three major types of diabetes namely type I, type II and gestational diabetes. According to senses taken in 2017, 8.8% of adult population worldwide was estimated to be diabetic which would shoot up to 9.9% by 2045,i.e about 6042 million of people would be affected worldwide. If diabetes is left untreated, it may lead to various diseases like kidney stone, diabetic retinopathy, diabetic neuropathy, stroke and heart attack. The people with diabetic neuropathy gradually lose sensitivity of the nervous system all over the body. Peripheral neuropathy is the most common type of diabetic neuropathy which is characterized by the loss of sensitivity in arms, hands, legs, feet and toes. If neuropathy in the foot is left untreated, it would increase the chances of occurrence of foot ulcers,

---

* Corresponding Authors' E-mail: arabi,punal@gmail.com, gayitrijoshi@gmail.com.

infection and amputation of the limb. To save the patients from these complications and to ensure the quality of the life of them, there is a need for early diagnosis.

This research work aims at proposing a non-invasive screening method for diabetes which is based on the thermoregulation of the peroneal vessel. Since diabetes affects the proneal vessel of the patients significantly, in this work the thermoregulatory behavior of peroneal vessel is studied for induced hot and cold stress. The study involved 20 subjects, out of which five persons are healthy or non-diabetic persons and the remaining 15 persons are of three categories namely patients with diabetes for less than 10 years, patients with diabetes for greater than 10 years, and patients with neuropathy; each category has five persons participating in this study.

The results obtained show the feasibility of disease screening by the proposed method although it is to be improved for further classification of the stages of disease progression and accuracy. From the results, it is seen that the thermoregulatory response of the peroneal blood vessel in the leg to the cold stress is more meaningful as a disease marker compared to hot stress. The accuracy of the proposed method is found be 75% for cold stress for a response time window of 2 minutes.

Keywords: machine vision, diabetes, neuropathy, thermoregulation, cold / hot stress

1. INTRODUCTION

Diabetes is a disease in which the body's ability to process blood glucose is impaired and the blood glucose, or blood sugar levels in the body are high. If this condition is left without careful management, then presence of too much of glucose in blood can cause serious problems over time. Diabetes can damage eyes, kidneys and nerves of a person and can also led to serious health problems like heart disease, stroke and diabetic neuropathy etc.

In the United States, it is estimated that 30.2 million of people over 18 years of age are suffering with diagnosed and undiagnosed diabetes; this figure is between 27.9% to 32.7% of the population. Though there are several types in diabetes, three types are the major ones namely Type 1, type 2, and gestational diabetes; managing the disease depends on the type.

Monogenic diabetes and cystic fibrosis-related diabetes are the less common types of diabetes.

1.1. Types

1.1.1. Type 1 Diabetes

When the body fails to produce insulin, type-1 diabetes also known as juvenile diabetes occurs. People with type-I diabetes must take artificial insulin daily to be alive.

1.1.2. Type 2 Diabetes

Type 2 diabetes is the most common type of diabetes. In this type the body does not produce enough insulin or use it effectively.

Type 1 diabetes and type 2 diabetes are chronic.

1.1.3. Gestational Diabetes

Gestational diabetes occurs in women during pregnancy and usually resolves after giving birth.

1.1.4. Pre Diabetes

Pre diabetes or borderline diabetes is the condition in which the blood sugar level is in the range of 100 to 125 milligrams per deciliter (mg/dL). The normal blood sugar level lies between 70 and 99 mg/dL where as for a person with diabetes fasting blood sugar level is higher than 126 mg/dL. People with pre diabetes have the risk of developing type 2 diabetes.

1.1.5. Symptoms

Diabetes symptoms vary depending on the elevation of blood sugar level. People with pre diabetes and type 2 diabetes may not experience any symptom initially. Symptoms of type 2 diabetes develop over many years. In type 1 diabetes, symptoms tend to develop in few weeks and would be severe.

Following are some of the symptoms of type 1 and type 2 diabetes:

- Increased thirst
- Frequent urination
- Extreme hunger
- Unexplained weight loss
- Presence of ketones in the urine
- Fatigue
- Irritability
- Blurred vision
- Slow-healing sores
- Frequent infections, such as gums or skin infections and vaginal infections

1.2. Causes

1.2.1. Type 1 Diabetes

In type -1diabetes, the cells of the pancreas which produce insulin are destroyed by the immune system.

This is an autoimmune condition and causes diabetes since the body does not have enough insulin to function normally.

Though there are no specific causes to be named, the following can be listed as risk factors:

- Viral or bacterial infection
- Chemical toxins within food
- Unidentified component causing autoimmune reaction
- Genetic

1.2.2. Type 2 Diabetes

Type 2 diabetes is caused usually by many factors with the family history being the main one.

The risk factors for type 2 diabetes are,

- Obesity
- Living a sedentary lifestyle
- Increasing age
- Bad diet
- The risk factors for pre diabetes are similar to type 2 diabetes.

1.3. Gestational Diabetes

The following are known to be the risk factors for gestational diabetes

- Family history of gestational diabetes
- Overweight or obese
- polycystic ovary syndrome
- Have had a large baby weighing over 9lb

The well-being of diabetic patients depends on the disease management which in turn depends on early diagnosis and treatment. This work describes a computer aided method for screening and diagnosis of diabetes using the thermoregulatory impairment of peroneal artery of the subjects.

2. LITERATURE SURVEY

Diabetes is one among the major health challenges of this century and is a serious, chronic but manageable disease. Most common method for estimation of blood glucose concentration is done by using glucose meters. The process involves pricking the finger and the blood extracted undergoes chemical analysis with the help of disposable test strips.

Daniela Matei. et al. [1] proposed a method using nerve conduction velocity of peripheral arterial disease(PAD) affected patients with and without diabetes mellitus (DM) for detecting and Characterizing peripheral neuropathy and also to find out if the degree of peripheral vascular impairment is consistent with the extent of nervous impairment.

Carla Agurto.et al. [2] developed a method based on cold stress provocation experiments using a cold patch and IR camera to obtain non-linear thermoregulation properties of the foot to detect diabetic peripheral neuropathy.

Punal M Arabi.et al. [3] presented a novel method to diagnose the foot impairment of diabetic patients using NIR imager and thermoregulatory behavior diabetic foot in which the NIR and the thermal images were statistically analyzed using pixel intensity matrix parameters.

K A Unnikrishna Menon.et al. [4] proposed a voltage intensity based non-invasive blood glucose monitoring method which is based on the principle of occlusion; in this method near infrared (NIR) light is passed through the fingertip before and after blocking the blood flow and the variations in voltage received after reflection are analyzed.

By analyzing the variation in voltages received after reflection in both the cases with the dataset, the current diabetic condition as well as the approximate glucose level of the individual is predicted.

Marti Widya Sari.et al. [5] discussed the design and analysis of a non-invasive blood glucose monitoring application to measure blood glucose levels in the body.

Haider Ali. et al. [6] introduced a method that uses a simple, compact and cost-effective non- invasive device using visible red laser light of wavelength 650 nm for blood glucose monitoring(RL-BGM). This method prevents the painful process of repetitive finger pricking and eliminates the risk of infection in diabetic patients.

K. Ammer P. Melnizky. et al. [7] investigated the occurrence of inverted thermal gradients in type 1 diabetic patients and correlated the hot spots on their feet with callus formation, toe nail onychomycosis and foot arch and toe deformities.

This paper showed that for about half of type 2 diabetic patients present with increased temperatures of their feet, however no relationship could be established with skin changes and areas of elevated skin temperature. Thermal imaging does not identify the common skin changes found in the feet of diabetics.

Omar Abdeladl. et al. [8] proved that within tissues high levels of deoxygenated blood or venous blood accumulation indicates poor blood circulation and increased risk of ulceration and this condition is associated with peripheral arterial occlusive disease or diabetic foot ulceration which is found to be the most common cause for lower extremity amputation. A near infrared camera was built utilizing a Raspberry Pi 2.0 System in conjunction with optical filters and image analysis tools to detect venous blood in tissues using differences in optical spectra of oxygenated versus deoxygenated blood in the near infrared (NIR)region.

B. Gayathri.et al. [9] proposed non-invasive method for blood glucose monitoring using near infrared spectroscopy system. In this work, both linear regression and polynomial regression analysis are studied for developing an enhanced algorithm for estimation of glucose concentration using the scattering property of glucose molecules and the principle of photoplethysmography. Bum Ju Lee.et al. [10] that whether a combination of various anthropometric measures that are measured in a greater number of specific sites in the body can improve the predictive power of diagnosing type 2 diabetes, irrespective of additional information like blood tests and concluded affirmatively.

Mohammad Hasan [11] showed that major complications in diabetes, if detected at the subclinical stage can be effectively treated and further complications can be avoided. The aim of this paper is to analyze the changes in the mechanical function of the ventricles in terms of systolic-diastolic interval interaction (SDI) from a surface ECG to assess the severity of CAN progression.

Nurhazwani Anang.et al. [12] analyzed the gait pattern of hip, knee, and ankle angles for stroke subjects diagnosed with diabetic peripheral neuropathy (DPN) and compared it with stroke subjects in order to identify diabetic peripheral neuropathy.

Geshwaree Huzooree. et al. [13] proposed a glucose prediction model using ARx to perform data analytics for a wireless body area network system.

Giovanni Mezzina. et al. [14] described the architecture of a wearable, wireless embedded system for diabetic peripheral neuropathy assessments in ordinary dynamic movements such as fluid gait. The proposed system implements a low computational complexity solution of the cross-correlation method using bitstream comparison between two EMGs on the same leg.

3. METHODOLOGY

The proposed method describes a computer aided screening procedure for diabetes. This work was carried out at Jnana Sanjeevini Diabetes Center, JP Nagar, Bangalore. The identified subjects signed an informed concerned form.

20 subjects participated in the study with five healthy non diabetic persons and in the remaining 15, five were in each category as patients with diabetes for less than 10 years, patients with diabetes for greater than 10 years and patients with neuropathy who had less or no sensation in the foot region. The subjects are asked to sit in the imaging room for 15 minutes to get acclimatized; the area of interest (Calf region) is cleaned as a part of pre imaging procedure. The cold/hot stress is then applied.

3.1. Cold Stress Experiment

The calf region is chosen as the area of interest since it is aimed to study the thermoregulatory impairment of peroneal artery with diabetes.

A cold stress using a cold pack at 0°C was applied to the calf muscle where the peroneal artery runs; the pack was kept for duration of 45 seconds after that it was removed. The temperature values of the calf were noted using a thermal imager as one image for every 20 seconds for a duration of 2 minutes. During this period due to thermoregulatory response of the subject's body, the calf area under test would try to heat up towards the temperature of the body. This procedure was repeated for all the subjects under observation. The corresponding temperature values were noted. Temperature values noted during the heating period of the calf area were compared and analysed. From the observed temperature values, ΔT value was calculated for every subject as

ΔT = Initial temperature (i.e., temperature at 0th sec) – temperature at 120th sec.

ΔT Avg, the average of all ΔT values for the subjects under observations was obtained and analysed.

3.2. Hot Stress Experiment

The same calf region is chosen as the area of interest for hot stress experiment also.

A hot stress using hot water bag at 45-50°C was applied to the calf muscle where the peroneal artery runs; the pack was kept for duration of 45 seconds after which it was removed. The temperature values of the calf were noted using a thermal imager as one image for every 20 seconds for a duration of 2 minutes. During this period due to thermoregulatory response of the subject's body the calf area under test would try to cool down towards the original temperature of the body. This producer was repeated for all the subjects. The corresponding temperature values were noted. Temperature values noted during the heating period of the calf area were compared and analysed. From the observed temperature values, ΔT value was calculated for every subject as

ΔT = Initial temperature – temperature at 120th sec.

ΔT Avg, the average of all ΔT values for the subjects under observation was obtained and analysed.

Figure1 shows the flow diagram of the proposed method.

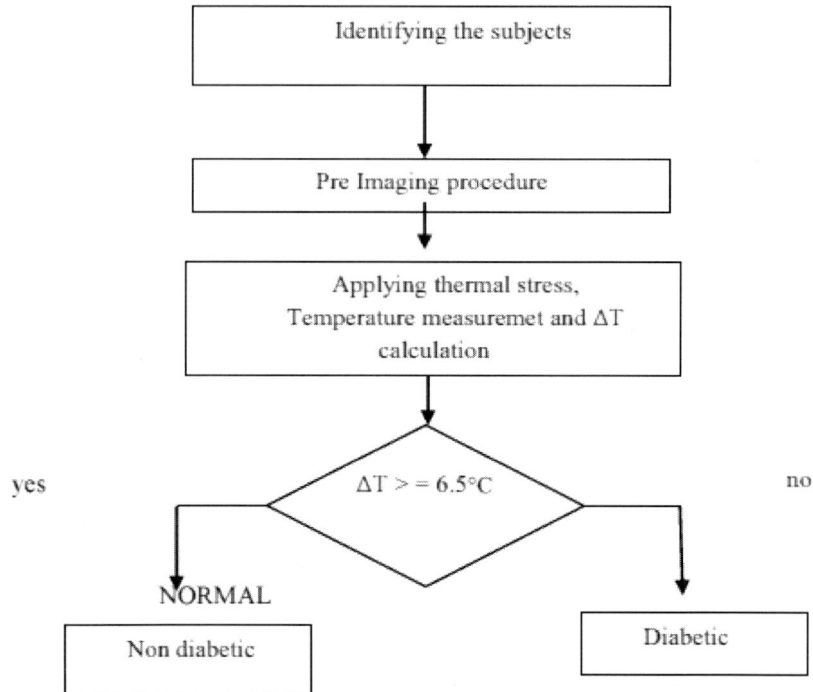

Figure 1. Proposed method.

4. RESULTS

Tables 1, 2, 3 and 4 show the patient data of age and sex. Tables 5,6,7 and 8 show the cold stress impact on thermoregulation of peroneal blood vessel of non diabetic and diabetic subjects with <10 years, >10 years of disease progression and diabetic neuropathy patients.

Tables 9,10,11 and 12 show the hot stress impact on thermoregulation of peroneal blood vessel of non diabetic and diabetic subjects with <10 years, >10 years of disease progression and diabetic neuropathy patients.

Figures 2 and 3 show the sample thermal images obtained by cold and hot stress experiments.

4.1. Patient Database

Table 1. Healthy Individuals

S.NO	Patient identification	Age	Sex
1	H1	63	Female
2	H2	51	Female
3	H3	46	Female
4	H4	83	Male
5	H5	66	Female

Table 2. Diabetic patients (<10 years)

S.NO	Patient identification	Age	Sex
1	P1	72	Male
2	P2	69	Male
3	P3	51	Female
4	P4	47	Male
5	P5	73	Female

Table 3. Diabetic patients (>10 YEARS)

S.NO	Patient identification	Age	Sex
1	P6	65	Female
2	P7	52	Male
3	P8	64	Female
4	P9	47	Female
5	P10	71	Male

Table 4. Diabetic neuropathy patients

S.NO	Patient identification	Age	Sex
1	P11	30	Male
2	P12	36	Female
3	P13	56	Female
4	P14	56	Female
5	P15	65	Female

4.2. Cold Stress

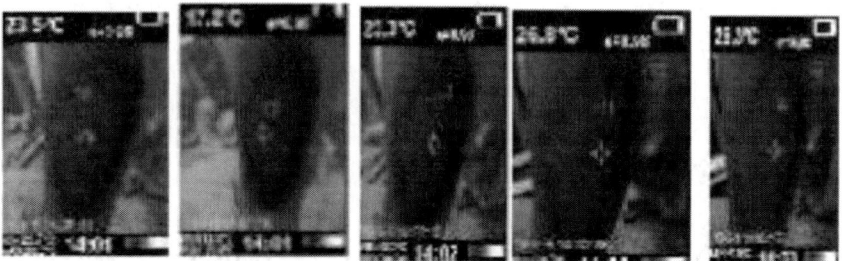

Figure 2. sample images of cold stress experiment.

Table 5. Non Diabetic Subjects - Cold Stress Impact on Peroneal Vessel

Subjects	Initial temp. ^{0}C	0th sec-temp ^{0}C	20th sec-temp. ^{0}C	40th sec-temp. ^{0}C	60th sec temp ^{0}C	80th sec temp^0 C	100th sec temp^0 C	120th sec temp^0 C	ΔT ^{0}C
H1	35.9	11	16.5	19.4	20.9	21.7	23.6	23.1	12.8
H2	34.4	28.7	26.5	29	29.6	30.7	30.7	31.8	2.6
H3	35.7	20.1	22.2	23.7	24.3	25.3	26.2	27.1	8.6
H4	35	21.5	25.6	26.4	27.1	28.4	28.7	29	6
H5	34.1	13.5	18.5	20.6	20.6	22.5	23.4	24.6	9.5
ΔT Avg									7.9

Table 6. Diabetic Subjects (<10 Years)-Cold Stress Impact on Peroneal Vessel

Subjects	Initial temp	0th sec temp ^{0}C	20th sec temp ^{0}C	40th sec temp ^{0}C	60th sec temp ^{0}C	80th sec temp ^{0}C	100th sec temp ^{0}C	120th sec temp^0 C	ΔT ^{0}C
P1	31.7	23.2	23.2	25.6	26	26.9	27.8	28.1	3.6
P2	36	28.3	31.3	32.9	33.2	34.1	34.5	33.6	2.4
P3	34.7	17.2	21.4	23.5	25.3	26.8	27.4	28.3	6.4
P4	36.9	27.4	28.1	29.1	29.1	29.5	31.2	31.7	5.2
P5	35	26.7	28.6	26.1	27.1	28.1	27.4	27.4	7.6
ΔT Avg									5.04

Table 7. Diabetic Subjects (>10 Years)-Cold Stress Impact On Peroneal Vessel

Subjects	Initial temp	0th sec Temp °C	20th sec temp° C	40th sec Temp °C	60th sec Temp °C	80th sec Temp °C	100th sec Temp °C	120th sec temp° C	ΔT °C
P6	*36.5*	29.8	28.2	30.9	31	32.2	32.1	32.8	3.7
P7	*34.8*	22.6	25.7	26.3	27.9	28.8	26.2	27.6	7.2
P8	*36*	27.6	27.6	27	28.5	29.5	30.1	30.4	5.6
P9	*34.8*	21.1	24.4	26.2	26.5	27.1	27.4	28.3	6.5
P10	*31.8*	20.2	24.3	31	29.3	29.5	26.8	29.8	2
ΔT Avg									5

Table 8. Neropathy Patients- Cold Stress Impact on Peroneal Vessel

Subjects	Initial Temp° C	0th sec Temp° C	20th sec temp° C	40th sec temp° C	60th sec temp° C	80th sec temp° C	100th sec temp° C	120th sec temp° C	ΔT °c
P11	*36.2*	21.5	25	26.2	26.2	27.1	27.7	27.7	8.5
P12	*36.5*	20	23.3	26.3	27.2	28.6	29.2	30.1	6.4
P13	*34.3*	20.8	26.1	26.7	27.6	28.2	29.2	29.5	4.8
P14	*35*	24.4	27.4	28.3	30.5	30.8	31.1	31.1	3.9
P15	*31.2*	29	29.3	29.6	30.3	30.3	30.3	30.3	0.9
ΔT Avg									4.9

4.3. Hot Stress

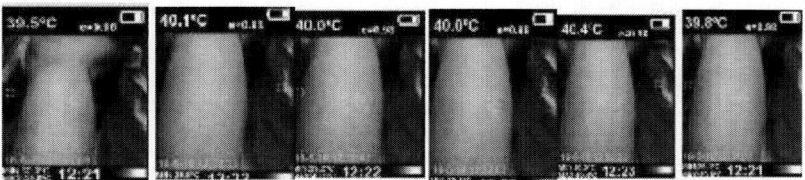

Figure 3. sample images of hot stress.

Table 9. Non-Diabetic Subjects - Hot Stress Impact on Peroneal Vessel

Subjects	Initial temp.	0th sec Temp °c	20th sec temp °c	40th sec temp °c	60th sec Temp °c	80th sec Temp °c	100th sec Temp °c	120th sec Temp °c	ΔT °c
S1	37.2	42.1	41.7	40.6	40.3	40.3	40	39.7	2.5
S2	35.2	41.9	40.5	40	39.3	39.4	39.4	39.4	4.2
S3	36	42	40.8	40.1	39.8	39.2	38.6	38.9	2.9
S4	34.8	38.3	37.4	36.5	35.4	35	34.1	34.1	0.7
S5	34.2	45.2	43.7	42.7	41.5	41.5	41.1	40.6	6.4
ΔT AVG									3.34

Table 10. Diabetic Subjects (<10 years) - Hot Stress Impact on Peroneal Vessel

Subjects	Initial temp.	0th sec temp °c	20th sec temp °c	40th sec temp °c	60th sec temp °c	80th sec Temp °c	100th sec Temp °c	120th sec Temp °c	ΔT °c
P1	37.7	42.3	39.2	38.9	38.3	38	37.7	37.1	0.6
P2	35.5	41.3	40.4	39.8	39.2	38.3	38.3	38	2.5
P3	40.5	48.7	45.6	44.7	43.4	42.5	43.2	41.5	1
P4	35.2	40.1	38.5	38.2	37.9	37.9	37.6	37.9	2.7
P5	36.2	45.2	43.7	42.7	41.5	41.5	41.1	40.6	4.4
ΔT AVG									2.24

Table 11. Diabetic Subjects (> 10 Years) - Hot Stress Impact on Peroneal Vessel

Subjects	Initial temp °c	0th sec Temp °c	20th sec Temp °c	40th sec Temp °c	60th sec Temp °c	80th sec Temp °c	100th sec Temp °c	120th sec Temp °c	ΔT °c
P6	33.5	42.9	41.1	40.5	40.2	39.2	38.9	38.9	5.4
P7	36.9	45.5	44.4	43.5	42.3	42.5	42.2	41.6	4.7
P8	36.3	43.7	42.9	42.9	41.6	40.3	41.2	40	3.7
P9	34.8	41.9	41.3	40.7	40.8	39.7	38.1	37.2	2.4
P10	33.4	45.2	44.8	44.2	43.8	42.9	42.4	41.4	8
ΔTAVG									4.84

Table 12. Neuropathy Patients - Hot Stress Impact on Peroneal Vessel

Subjects	Initial temp. °c	0th sec temp °c	20th sec Temp °c	40th sec Temp °c	60th sec Temp °c	80th sec Temp °c	100th sec temp °c	120th sec Temp °c	ΔT °c
P11	*35.9*	38.8	38.9	38	38.3	37.7	38.1	37.8	1.9
P12	*41.4*	47.5	45.3	43.9	44.2	43.8	43.2	43.2	1.8
P13	*39.2*	48.5	45.9	44.7	43.8	43.5	43.2	42.3	3.1
P14	*34.7*	40.3	39	38.4	37.8	37.2	36.9	36.6	1.9
5 P1	*31.7*	42.3	42.1	41.7	**41.7**	40.6	**39.3**	37.1	5.4
ΔT AVG									2.82

5. DISCUSSION

A noninvasive method based on the thermoregulatory response of the peroneal blood vessel in the leg is proposed for screening of diabetes. The thermoregulatory response is induced by the application of hot or cold stress. The temperature variations produced by the induced thermoregulatory response are noted and tabulated. From the tabulated results, it is seen that the thermoregulatory response of the peroneal blood vessel in the leg to the cold stress are more meaningful compared to hot stress for a response time window of 2 minutes.

From Table-5, it is seen that $\Delta T = 7.9\ ^0$ C for non diabetics for an observation window of 2 minutes by cold stress application. For diabetic patients with disease progression >10 years, <10 years and neuropathy, ΔT is found to be 5.04^0 C, 5^0 C, 4.9^0 C from tables 6, 7 and 8 respectively. From these values the threshold value is calculated as

$$\Delta T_T = [7.9 + (5.04+5+4.9)/3]/2\ ^0 C$$
$$= (7.9+4.98)/2\ ^0 C$$
$$= 6.5^0 C$$

where ΔT_T is the threshold value.

Based on the threshold value the decision rule is framed for diabetes screening.

For classifying diabetics and non-diabetics, the change in temperature ΔT_T is considered and if $\Delta T_T > 6.5\ °c$, the subject is classified as non-diabetic; otherwise the subject is diabetic.

From Table-9, it is seen that $\Delta T = 3.34\ ^0C$ for non-diabetics for an observation window of 2 minutes by hot stress application. For diabetic patients with disease progression >10 years, <10 years, neuropathy ΔT is found to be 2.24^0C, 4.84^0C, 2.82^0C from tables 10, 11 and 12 respectively. Hence these values do not yield any useful finding, the hot stress impact could not be analysed at this level.

CONCLUSION

The proposed method is a non-invasive method to diagnose diabetes which is based on the thermoregulation of the peroneal artery. Out of 20 subjects taken for analysis, 5 were healthy and 15 were diabetes at different stages of disease progression. Out 20 subjects taken for experimentation, 15 answered the decision rule. Out of the 5subjects which did not answer the decision rule, 2 non-diabetic subjects were identified as diabetic and 3 diabetic subjects were identified as non-diabetic. Hence accuracy of the proposed method is 75% with 10% false positive and 15% false negative.

The proposed method shows the feasibility of machine vision for screening and early diagnosis of diabetes using the thermoregulatory impairment of peroneal blood vessel. However, it is to be improved for further classification of stages of disease progression and accuracy.

REFERENCES

[1] Daniela Matei, Cálin Corciová, Radu Matei, "Nerve Conduction Studies in Peripheral Arterial Disease With and Without Type 2

Diabetes Mellitus", *2013 E-Health and Bioengineering Conference (EHB)*, 1-4, 2013, https://doi.org/10.1109/ehb.2013.6707331.

[2] Carla Agurto, Viktor Chek, Ana Edwards, Zyden Jarry, Simon Barriga, Janet Simon, Peter Soliz, "A thermoregulation model to detect diabetic peripheral neuropathy", *South West Symposium on Image Analysis and Interpretation*, pp.13-16,IEEE(2016).

[3] Punal M. Arabi; Surekha Nigudgi, Tejaswi Bhat; Abrar Ahmed, "Investigations on diabetic foot impairment using NIR images and thermoregulatory behavior", *2017 8th International Conference on Computing, Communication and Networking Technologies (ICCCNT)*, pp-1-5,IEEE(2017).

[4] K. A. Unnikrishna Menon, Deepak Hemachandran; Abishek Thekkeyil Kunnat, "Voltage intensity based non-invasive blood glucose monitoring," *2013 Fourth International Conference on Computing, Communications and Networking Technologies (ICCCNT)*, pp-1-5,IEEE(2013), DOI: 10.1109/ICCCNT.2013. 6726720.

[5] Marti Widya Sari,Muhtar Luthfi, "Design and analysis of non-invasive blood glucose levels monitoring", *2016 International Seminar on Application for Technology of Information and Communication (ISemantic)* pp. 134-137.doi: 10.1109/ISEMANTIC. 2016.7873825.

[6] Haider Ali, Faycal Bensaali, Fadi Jaber, "Novel approach to non invasive blood glucose monitoring based on transmittance and refraction of visible laser light" pp- 9163 – 9174, *IEEE* (2017) DOI: 10.1109/ACCESS.2017.2707384.

[7] K. Ammer P. Melnizky 2, 0. Rathkolb 2, E.F. Ring, "Thermal Imaging of Skin Changes on the Feet of Type I1 Diabetics", *2001 Proceedings of the 23rd Annual EMBS International Conference*, pp. 2870-2872, IEEE (2001).

[8] Omar Abdeladl, Michelle Schleicher, Margarita Portilla; Aleksey Shaporev; Vladimir Reukov, "Development of a Portable Near Infrared Camera for Early Detection of Diabetic Ulcers", *2016 32nd*

Southern *Biomedical Engineering Conference (SBEC)*, DOI: 10. 1109/SBEC.2016.73, pp-55-56,IEEE(2016).

[9] B. Gayathri K. Sruthi; K. A. Unnikrishna Menon, "Non-invasive blood glucose monitoring using near infrared spectroscopy", *2017 International Conference on Communication and Signal Processing (ICCSP)*, DOI: 10.1109/ICCSP.2017.8286555, pp. 1139-1142, IEEE (2017)

[10] Bum Ju Lee, Boncho Ku, Jiho Nam, Duong Duc Pham, and Jong Yeol Kim, "Prediction of Fasting Plasma Glucose Status Using Anthropometric Measures for Diagnosing Type 2 Diabetes", *IEEE Journal of Biomedical and Health Informatics*, vol. 18, NO. 2, March 2014, pp. (555-561)

[11] Mohammad Hasan Imam, Chandan K. Karmakar, Herbert F. Jelinek, Marimuthu Palaniswami, and Ahsan H. Khandoker, "Analyzing Systolic–Diastolic Interval Interaction Characteristics in Diabetic Cardiac Autonomic Neuropathy Progression", *IEEE Journal of Translational Engineering in Health and Medicine,* volume 3, (IEEE), 2015, DOI:10.1109/JTEHM.2015.2462339,pp-1900510.

[12] Nurhazwani Anang, Rozita Jailani, Nooritawati Md Tahir,Haidzir Manaf, Nadia Mustafah, "Analysis of Kinematic Gait Parameters in Stroke with Diabetic Peripheral Neuropathy (DPN)", *2016 IEEE Conference on Systems, Process and Control (ICSPC 2016)*, 16–18 December 2016, Melaka, Malaysia.pp.136-141.

[13] Geshwaree Huzooree,Kavi Kumar Khedo, Noorjehan Joonas, "Glucose Prediction Data Analytics for Diabetic patients Monitoring", *2017 1st International Conference on Next Generation Computing Applications (NextComp)*, pp-1-8, IEEE(2017), DOI: 10.1109/NEXTCOMP.2017.8016197.

[14] Giovanni Mezzina, Vito Leonardo Gallo, Daniela De Venuto, "Real-Time Muscle Fiber Conduction Velocity Tracker for Diabetic Neuropathy Monitoring", *2017 7th IEEE International Workshop on Advances in Sensors and Interfaces (IWASI)*, pp-1-6, IEEE(2017, doi: 10.1109/iwasi.2017.7974232.

In: Diabetic Foot: Prevention and Treatment ISBN: 978-1-53616-266-0
Editor: Gianni Romano © 2019 Nova Science Publishers, Inc.

Chapter 2

CLINICAL APPLICATIONS OF MESENCHYMAL STEM CELLS IN NON-HEALING DIABETIC FOOT ULCERS (DFUs): AN EFFECTIVE TREATMENT

Surjya Narayan Dash[1,3,*], *Nihar Ranjan Dash*[1,2] *and Prakash Chandra Mohapatra*[1,4] *

[1]Department of Biochemistry, SCB Medical College Cuttack, Odisha. India
[2]Department of Biochemistry, Apollo Hospitals Bhubaneswar, Odisha. India
[3]Institute of Biotechnology, University of Helsinki, Finland
[4]Regional Spinal Injury Center, SCB Medical College Campus, Cuttack Odisha, India

ABSTRACT

Diabetes Mellitus is the condition where the level of sugar in blood is high. There are many complications of diabetes, Diabetic Foot Ulcer

---

* Corresponding Authors' E-mails: drpcmohapatra@gmail.com; surjya.dash30@gmail.com.

(DFU) being one of the most common complications of long-standing diabetes. Majority of the patients with diabetes foot ulcer (DFU) advance to amputations. DFU has emerged as one of the leading causes of mortality and morbidity and has a great financial implication on individual and the society. Therapeutic application of autologous BM-derived Mesenchymal stem cells (MSCs) have revolutionized the field of regenerative medicine and emerged as a promising therapeutic strategy to treat DFU. MSCs have multi-lineage differentiation potential and upon implantation they secrete cytokines that promote cell recruitment, immunomodulation, extracellular matrix remodeling, angiogenesis, and neuroregeneration facilitating wound healing. However, more detailed clinical studies and post-implantation follow up is required before it is used as cell replacement therapy (CRT) for nonhealing ulcers of the lower extremities in a larger context. This chapter highlights recent findings in the areas of hMSCs (human MSCs) sources, its differentiation ability, immunogenicity, adaptation to the microenvironment by secreting paracrine factors and its use in human clinical trials in DFUs.

Keywords: diabetes, foot ulcer, wound healing, bone marrow, mesenchymal stem cells

1. Diabetes Mellitus

1.1. Introduction to Diabetes Mellitus

Diabetes mellitus is a condition characterized by increase in blood sugar as a result of loss of the body's capability to utilize blood sugar. The term Diabetes mellitus was coined from-. '*diabetes*' the Greek word meaning 'siphon' or to pass through and '*mellitus*' the Latin word meaning 'honeyed' or sweet. To understand diabetes, we have to understand the use of glucose in the body and the role of insulin in glucose metabolism. Sugar is the source of energy for the body to perform various activity. The food that we take contains sugar (in form of carbohydrates and starch) along with other nutrients. The process of digestion begins in the mouth itself and is completed by the time the food reaches the small intestine. Our stomach plays a vital role in the process of digestion. When the stomach digests food, all forms of sugar present as carbohydrate and starch in the food breaks down into simple sugar, called glucose. The small intestines absorb the glucose and then release it into the bloodstream. Once in the bloodstream, glucose can be used immediately for energy or stored in our body, to be used it later.

The cells in the body utilize the sugar in form of glucose to derive energy for daily activities. To be utilized sugar cannot enter the cells by itself. The beta cells of the pancreas releases insulin into the blood, which facilitates the entry of sugar across the cell membrane into the cells. When sugar leaves the bloodstream and enters the cells, the blood sugar level is lowered in the bloodstream. Without insulin sugar cannot get into the body's cells and this causes blood sugar to rise resulting in a condition called Diabetes Mellitus. Insulin also stimulates the liver to absorb and store any excess glucose in blood. Insulin release is triggered after a meal when there is a rise in blood glucose.

1.2. Classification of Diabetes

There are two main types of diabetes: type 1 and type 2: Type 1 diabetes occurs because the insulin-producing cells of the pancreas (beta-cells) are damaged. This was previously known as insulin-dependent, juvenile or childhood-onset diabetes. In type 1 diabetes, the pancreas makes little or no insulin, so sugar cannot be used as energy source. It is characterized by deficient insulin production and requires daily administration of insulin. Though Type 1 is most commonly seen in people below the age of 30 years, it can occur in any age group. Ten percent of people with diabetes are diagnosed with type 1 (Diagnosis and classification of diabetes mellitus. Diab care. 2009; 32 (Suppl 1): S62–S67 (American diabetes association).

Type 2 diabetes, previously called as non-insulin-dependent, or adult-onset diabetes occurs when the pancreas makes insulin, but it either doesn't produce enough, or the insulin does not work properly. This type occurs most often in people who are over 40 years old but can occur even in childhood with the presence of risk factors. 90 percent of people with diabetes have type- 2 (Definition, diagnosis and classification of diabetes mellitus and its complications. Part 1: Diagnosis and classification of diabetes mellitus. WHO/NCD/NCS/99.2. Geneva: World Health Organization; 1999).

1.3. Prevalence of Diabetes

World Health Organization (WHO) data shows that number of diabetic patients increased from 108 million in 1980 to 422 million in 2014.The global prevalence of diabetes among adults over 18 years of age has risen from 4.7% in 1980 to 8.5% in 2014 (Swar et al. 2010). In 2015, 30.3 million Americans, or 9.4% of the population, had diabetes. In 2017, there were 425 million people with diabetes worldwide, out of which 82 million people in the were South East Asia Region; and by 2045 this number is estimated to rise to 151 million. In India 72,946,400 cases of diabetes (8.8% of adult population) reported in 2017. Diabetes emerged as India's seventh biggest cause of early death in 2016, up from 11th in 2005. Around 47.3% of India's 70 million are undiagnosed diabetic patients. 12% of the global health expenditure is spent on treating diabetes and its related complications as per International Diabetes Federation estimation (US$ 673 billion). According to a report by Pricewater house Coopers, if we go by the current treatment costs, India's total bill for treating diabetes would be US$30 billion by 2025. But with economic growth and standards of care improving, treatment costs are likely to rise, and it has been estimated the same cost to go up to US$79.7 billion. Diabetes prevalence has risen more rapidly in middle- and low-income countries.

1.4. Complications due to Diabetes

Due to lack or insufficiency of insulin high blood glucose is observed in diabetes patients. Excess glucose in the blood can damage the blood vessels and can affect several organs like the heart, kidneys and eyes.

Uncontrolled Diabetes increases the likelihood of infections. Infections and gangrene of the lower limbs may need an amputation if severe. People with diabetes are also 15 per cent more likely to go for amputation than people without the condition (Moxey et al., 2011). Long-term complications of diabetes develop gradually. Longer the duration of diabetes the higher is the risk of complications. Eventually, diabetic complications may be disabling or even life-threatening. Possible complications include:

1.4.1. Cardiovascular Disease

Diabetes increases the risk of various cardiovascular problems. This may contribute to coronary artery disease with narrowing of arteries (atherosclerosis), chest pain and angina. Adults with history of diabetes have two- or three-times higher rate of cardiovascular disease (CVD) than adults without diabetes (Emerging Risk Factors Collaboration and Sarwar et al., 2010).

1.4.2. Nerve Damage (Neuropathy)

The mechanism of neuropathy is poorly understood. It is due to direct metabolic effect of hyperglycemia or secondary to hypoxia from microvascular involvement. As a result of increased flux in the polyol pathway secondary to hyperglycaemia, sorbitol accumulation causes decrease nerve conduction and membrane damage. Advanced Glycocylated End Products (AGEs) formed as a result of chronic hyperglycemis, also damage the nerves. Oxidative stress due to long-standing diabetes cause activation of cytokines and decrease the production of Nitric Oxide which further damage the nerve. There are four types of diabetic neuropathy: **Peripheral neuropathy** causes pain or loss of feeling in the hands, arms, feet, and legs. This is most common type of neuropathy seen in diabetic patients. **Autonomic neuropathy** can cause bowel and bladder dysfunction, difficulty in swallowing, and erectile dysfunction. It can also affect the nerves that control the heart and blood pressure. **Proximal neuropathy** causes weakness in the legs. **Focal neuropathy** can affect any nerve in the body, leading to pain or weakness.

1.4.3. Kidney Damage (Nephropathy)

The kidneys contain millions of tiny blood vessel clusters (glomeruli) that filter waste from the blood. Diabetes can damage this delicate filtering system. Glycosylation of glomerular proteins as a result of diabetes cause mesangial cell proliferation and vascular endothelial damage. The glomerular basement membrane classically becomes thickened and it is the hallmark of diabetic nephropathy. Severe damage can lead to kidney failure or irreversible end-stage kidney disease, which may need dialysis or a kidney transplant. The incidence of ESRD is up to 10 times as high in adults with diabetes as those without diabetes.

1.4.4. Eye Damage (Retinopathy)

Diabetes can damage the blood vessels of the retina (diabetic retinopathy), potentially leading to blindness. The mechanism of Diabetic retinopathy includes oxidative stress, advance glycosylation end products and increased polyol pathway flux. The hallmark of retinopathy includes loss of retinal capillary cells (pericytes and endothelial cells), basement membrane thickening, microaneurysms and vascular obstruction. Diabetes also increases the risk of other serious conditions, such as cataracts and glaucoma. Diabetic retinopathy caused 1.9% of moderate or severe visual impairment globally and 2.6% of blindness in 2010 (Bourne et al., 2013).

1.4.5. Foot Ulcers

Long standing diabetes result in damaged nerves and blood vessels of the lower limbs. Due to decreased sensation in the lower limbs, small cuts and wounds might go unnoticed. Reduced blood supply result in delayed healing which gets infected over a period of time. These infections may ultimately require toe, foot or leg amputation. Diabetes increases the risk of lower extremity amputation because of infected, non-healing foot ulcers.

1.4.6. Skin Conditions

Diabetes can affect every part of the body, counting the skin. Many people with diabetes will have a skin disorder caused or aggravated by diabetes at some point in their life. Long term diabetes damages the blood vessels and nerves of the skin resulting in changes in appearance, texture and healing capacity of the skin. In some cases, skin problems are the first sign that a person has diabetes. People with diabetes also are more prone to getting certain conditions. These include diabetic dermopathy, necrobiosis lipoidica diabeticorum, and eruptive xanthomatosis. Diabetes may increase the possibilities of skin problems like styes, boils, carbuncles, folliculitis and infections, including bacterial and fungal infections. It is estimated that one-third of people with diabetes will have some skin related problems.

1.4.7. Depression

Depression is common in people with type 1 and type 2 diabetes. Studies show that people with diabetes have a greater risk of depression than people without diabetes. Depression can affect diabetes management; Diabetes may lead to poor lifestyle decisions. Unhealthy eating, less exercise, smoking and weight gain — all of which are risk factors for diabetes.

2. DIABETIC FOOT ULCER (DFU)

2.1. Introduction to Diabetic Foot Ulcer (DFU)

Foot ulcers are the most common medical complications of patients with diabetes, with an estimated prevalence of 12-15% among all individuals with diabetes (American Diabetes Association: Diabetes statistics. Available at: www.diabetes.org/diabetes-statistics.jsp). The risk of developing a diabetic foot ulcer increases with time. Diabetic foot ulcers remain a major health care problem. Diabetes and its related complications cause high morbidity mortality as well as considerable financial burden. Several factors are involved in the decreased healing potential of a diabetic foot. The factors are: Level of uncontrolled hyperglycemia, Reduced circulation and arterial blood flow, Nutrition status, Inability to offload the affected region of the foot and Presence of infection (American Diabetes Association: Diabetes statistics. Available at: www.diabetes.org/diabetes-statistics.jsp). The etiology of diabetic foot ulcers is multifactorial, but minor trauma in the presence of peripheral sensory neuropathy is the primary culprit. Peripheral neuropathy is present in 60% of patients with diabetes and 80% of patients with diabetes who have foot ulcers. Decreased sensation in the foot predisposes the patient with diabetes to unnoticed injuries and fractures that overload the skin and lead to ulceration. DFUs often require extensive healing time and are associated with increased risk for infections and other complications that can result in severe and costly outcomes (Frykberg et al., 2006). Studies have estimated that foot ulceration is one of the major sources of hospitalizations among patients with diabetes and precedes 84% of amputations of lower limbs in these patients (Pecoraro et al., 1990). In addition, DFU patients have a low survival prognosis, with a 3-year cumulative mortality rate of 28% (Margolis et al., 2013) and mortality rates among amputated patients approaching 50% (Armstrong et al., 2007).

2.2. Treatment of DFUs

International Best Practice Guidelines: Wound Management in Diabetic Foot Ulcers (International Best Practice Guidelines: Wound Management in Diabetic Foot Ulcers. Wounds International 2013). states that the most effective care of DFUs involves optimal diabetes control, effective local wound care, infection control, pressure relieving strategies, and optimization of blood flow. The current therapy options for DFUs include:

2.2.1. Debridement

Debridement is a mainstay of topical treatment for DFUs. It removes nonviable and infected tissue, old and worn out cells, pseudoepithelium and biofilms. Additionally, sharp debridement also stimulates neomicrovascular circulation. Mechanical debridement and wound lavage help in removing any bacterial contaminants and can assist in preventing colonization, or infection. It can also help stimulate neovascularization and healthy cell proliferation.

2.2.2. Autografts and Allografts

The use of split-thickness autografts in DFU treatment entails the transfer of fascia from a donor to the wound. Healing occurs in about 6 weeks and it is cosmetically pleasing, leaving only scarring and contracture around the wound. The most evident limitations are donor skin availability and the limited number of proliferating cells in donor skin (Dreifke et al., 2015). Currently available alternative skin grafting products include extracellular matrices; xenografts using porcine dermis, porcine intestinal submucosa, or bovine collagen; synthetic bilayer skin substitutes; acellular skin substitutes; cultured epidermal substitutes; neonatal immortalized keratinocytes; dermal substitutes using newborn foreskin fibroblast cells; and composite skin substitutes with a collagen scaffold, cultured fibroblasts, and stratified cultured keratinocytes

2.2.3. Offloading

Offloading options include total contact casts (TCCs), custom sandals, cast walkers, Charcot restraint orthotic walkers, braces, and ankle-foot orthoses. In patients with a high risk of recurrent ulcers and when traditional offloading methods have failed, surgical offloading is an alternative option.

3. WOUND HEALING AND CHRONIC WOUNDS

3.1. Wound Healing

Wound healing involves a series of immunologic and biological events resulting in closure of a wound. The normal healing process involves growth factor activation, cellular activity, and formation of connective tissue, which occur in an orderly and timely manner. If a wound does not heal in a timely and/or orderly fashion or if there is a loss of structural integrity, then the wound is considered chronic or non- healing wound. There are 3 phases of wound healing, namely-

3.1.1. Inflammatory Phase

This phase typically lasts for 24 hours. The inflammatory phase results in homeostasis and removal of debris from the site. The main cell types involved are the platelets and the WBCs (neutrophils and Macrophages). Injury cause initial release of epinephrine and intense vasoconstriction (within 5-10 minutes) to reduce blood loss, it is followed by release of inflammatory mediators (histamine, prostaglandins) from mast cells resulting in active vasodilation and increased capillary permeability (within 10-30 minutes). Now platelets attach to the exposed sub endothelial collagen surface. They form the initial platelet plug and get activated thereby secreting platelet-derived growth factor *(PDGF)*, proteases, and vasoactive amines (e.g., serotonin, histamine). The coagulation cascade occurs through two separate pathways, the intrinsic and the extrinsic pathway. The result of platelet aggregation and the coagulation cascade is clot formation.

Thrombin activated during clot formation facilitates migration of inflammatory cells to the site of injury by increasing vascular permeability. Factors and cells necessary to heal flow from the intravascular space into the extravascular space. Neutrophils enter the wound to fight infection and to attract macrophages. Macrophages break down necrotic debris and activate the fibroblast response.

3.1.2. Proliferative Phase

This phase typically lasts for 2- 21 days. This phase results in the formation of granulation tissue, angiogenesis, wound contraction and epithelialization. The main cell types involved are fibroblast, endothelial cells and keratinocytes. Fibroblasts proliferate in the deeper parts of the wound. These fibroblasts begin to synthesize small amounts of collagen which acts as a scaffold for migration and further fibroblast proliferation. Macrophages stimulate the fibroblasts to produce Glycosaminoglycans (GAGS) and immature collagen which improves wound tensile strength.

Macrophages also promote formation of new blood vessels from endothelial cells of damaged vessels (angiogenesis). Thus, granulation tissue, which consists of capillary loops supported in this developing collagen matrix, appears in the deeper layers of the wound in 24-72 hours.

Four to five days after the injury, fibroblasts begin producing large amounts of collagen and proteoglycans. Collagen fibers are laid down randomly and are cross-linked to increase the wound strength. Wound contraction starts in one week once wound is filled with granulation tissue. Some fibroblasts transform to smooth muscle actin (myofibroblasts) which moves wound edges closer. Wound re-epithelisation occurs when keratinocytes migrate across the wound, differentiate and form strata of neodermis.

3.1.3 Maturation Phase

This phase typically starts 3 weeks after injury and may continue up to 2 years. During the maturation phase, fibroblasts leave the wound and collagen is remodeled into a more organized matrix. Tensile strength increases for up to one year following the injury. Healed wounds can regain up to 70 to 80% of its original strength.

3.2. Chronic Wound

A chronic or non-healing wound does not progress normally through the wound healing process, resulting in an open wound. These conditions are caused by a number of pathophysiological conditions, which essentially lead to a hyper-inflammatory environment. In a chronic wound the healing process is stalled in the inflammatory phase.

All the three physiologic healing processes are altered in non-healing ulcers and contribute to poor healing. In a non-healing DFU, the following abnormalities are observed: decreased or impaired growth factor production, angiogenic response, macrophage function, collagen accumulation, epidermal barrier function, abnormal quantity of granulation tissue, keratinocyte and fibroblast migration and proliferation. The balance between accumulation of ECM components and their remodeling by matrix metalloproteinases (MMPs) is also altered. The final result of the above changes keeps the diabetic ulcer stuck in the inflammatory phase of the wound healing process. Under normal circumstances, this phase lasts only 2 – 3 days, followed by the proliferative phase and in wound closure. However, a DFU fails to progress to the proliferative phase and remains in a chronic inflammatory phase.

4. MESENCHYMAL STEM CELLS (MSCs)

4.1. Introduction to MSCs

Cell therapy based on stem cells refers to the process of introducing stem cells into the tissue to treat or prevent a disease or condition. Stem cells are unspecialized cells with the ability to renew themselves for long periods without significant changes in their general properties. They can differentiate into various specialized cell types with varied potency (Wei et al., 2013) under certain physiological or experimental conditions. Stem cells become a pronounced subject because of its importance in cell transplantation therapies and modern biological research era. On the basis of origin, stem cells are divided into different categories. Hematopoietic stem cells (HSCs) have been widely used for allogeneic cell therapy. The successful isolation of pluripotent embryonic stem (ES) cells from the inner cell mass of early embryos has provided a powerful tool for biological research. ES cells can give rise to almost all cell lineages and are the most promising cells for regenerative medicine. The ethical issues related to isolation have promoted the development of induced pluripotent stem (iPS) cells, which share many properties with ES cells without ethical concerns. However, one key property of ES cells and iPS cells that may seriously compromise their utility is their potential for teratoma formation. Researcher around the world are looking for safe and stable stem cell sources that can be used for therapeutically application. Mesenchymal stem cells (MSCs) are multipotent stromal cells that can differentiate into a variety of cell types, including osteoblasts (bone cells), chondrocytes (cartilage cells), myocytes (muscle cells) and adipocytes (fat cells which give rise to marrow adipose tissue). Mesenchymal stem cells isolated from mouse bone marrow differentiate into specialized cells types, exhibiting the property of adherence and formed spindle-shaped colonies, and were referred as colony forming unit fibroblasts (Friedenstein et al., 1976). MSCs exists in different adult tissues possess self-renewal while maintaining their multipotency properties with genomic stability.*In vitro* they can be expanded with limited ethical issues, marking its importance in cell therapy, and tissue repair (Horwitz et al., 2015). The standard steps to confirm multipotency of MSCs is by differentiating them into osteoblasts, adipocytes and chondrocytes as well as myocytes and neurons.

4.2. Sources of Mesenchymal Stem Cells

There are several sources from where MSCs can be isolated. MSC originating from the bone marrow (BM) are gold standards, the most commonly used stem cells in clinical trials compared to other sources. Most stem cells isolated either from the patient's bone marrow or from adipose tissue are intended for cell-based therapies. These cells are induced to differentiate exclusively into the adipocytic, chondrocytic, or osteocytic lineages (Pittenger et al., 1999). These adult stem cells could be individually identified and expanded to colonies, retaining their multilineage potential. Cells exhibiting characteristics of MSCs are isolated from adipose tissue (Wagner et al., 2005). Amniotic fluid is an abundant source of fetal MSCs that exhibit phenotype and multilineage differentiation potential (In'tAnker et al., 2003). Five different types of human dental stem/progenitor cells have been characterized, dental pulp stem cells (DPSCs), stem cells from exfoliated deciduous teeth (SHED), periodontal ligament stem cells (PDLSCs), stem cells from apical papilla (SCAP), and dental follicle progenitor cells (DFPCs) (Huang et al., 2009). All of these possess mesenchymal-stem-cell-like (MSC) qualities, including the capacity for self-renewal and multilineage differentiation.

Characteristic features of stem cells include long-term culturing properties; differentiation into multiple cell types, clonality; expression of markers CD146, CD105, CD90, CD73, MSI1, NOTCH1, and SOX2; and absence of CD34 and CD14 expression (Schuring et al., 2011). Allickson et al., (2011) identified the proliferative capability and multilineage potential of stem cells in menstrual blood. Similarly, differentiation of MSC (adherent) and HSC (suspension), from peripheral blood into osteoblast (MSC) and osteoclast (HSC) are assessed (Kadir et al., 2012). Use of extra embryonic mesenchymal stem cells found in the umbilical cord, yolk sac and placenta and testing their differentiating capabilities are the recent new areas of interest. These stem cells possess higher differentiating ability than the adult counterparts, including the ability to more readily form tissues of endodermal and ectodermal origin. Fetal-tissue are considered as a major source of MSCs. MSCs isolated from fresh placenta (Pl-MSC) and fetal membrane (Mb-MSC) shows higher osteogenic differentiation potential, their comparative analysis shows Pl-MSC performance is better (Raynaud et al., 2012). Mesenchymal stem cells (MSCs) present in SF was reported previously (Morito, et al., 2008). Mesenchymal cells isolated from the umbilical cord express CD44, CD105 and integrin markers (CD29, CD51) but not hematopoietic lineage markers (CD34, CD45). Wharton's jelly of the umbilical cord contains mucoid connective tissue and fibroblast-like cells, interestingly mesenchymal stem cell markers (SH2, SH3) expression is significant in these cells (Wang et al., 2004). Mesenchymal stromal cells have been described and isolated from many different adult tissues (see Table-1), including bone marrow, adipose tissue, inner organs, and blood vessels and from sources such as amniotic fluid, amniotic membrane, umbilical cord, or placenta. In order to distinguish MSCs from the fibroblasts and other adherently growing cells, suitable cell surface markers of MSCs are the best option for cell sorting and implementing it in experiments. Research is ongoing to find new sources of mesenchymal stem cells present in the skin and dermis because easy availability with minimal risk (Park et al., 2012).

Table 1. Differentiation of MSCs into different cell Types from their sources

Bone marrow	Adipocyte, Astrocyte, Cardiomyocyte Chondrocyte, Hepatocyte, Mesangial cells Myocyte, Neuron, Osteoblast, Stromal cells
Adipose tissue	Chondrocyte, Myocyte, Osteoblast, Stromal cells
Muscle	Adipocyte, Endothelial cell, Neuron, Chondrocyte, Osteocyte
Dental pulp	Chondrocytes, Osteocytes, Adipocytes, Neuronal cells, Pancreatic cells, Melanocytes
Endometrium	Adipocytes, Chondrocytes, Osteoblasts
Synovial membrane	Adipocyte, Chondrocyte, Myocyte, Osteoblast
Blood	Osteoblast, Osteoclast, Adipocyte, Fibroblast
Pericytes	Chondrocytes
Trabecular bone	Osteoblast, Myocyte, Adipocyte, Chondrocyte
Periosteum	Osteoblast, Chondrocyte

4.3. Expression of Cell Surface Markers

The standard criteria set by International Society for Cellular Therapy suggest that expression of specific set cell surface markers is one of the essential characteristics of hMSCs. MSCs cells are positive for CD73, D90, CD105 and HLA-DR and negative expression for CD14, CD34, CD45. There are controversies in expression of cell surface markers for characterization of MSCs for example: MSCs derived from few specific tissues are positive for CD29, CD44, CD146, CD140b and negative for CD34, (Lin et al., 2012). Some studies suggest that stage-specific embryonic antigen (SSEA)-4 (Vaculik et al., 2012), CD146 (Zhang et al., 2011) and stromal precursor antigen-1 (Stro-1) (Park et al., 2011) are the stemness markers for MSCs. MSCs derived from human amniotic fluid express CD29, CD44, CD90, CD105 and HLA-ABC (major histocompatibility complex class I (MHC I)) along with SH2 (Src homology 2), SH3 (Src homology 3), SH4 (Src homology 4) but lack the expression of HLA-DR (MHC II) (Tsai et al., 2004). Stro-1, which is consider as stemnes marker for MSCs, is reported positive in dental pup (Kadar, et al., 2009) and bone marrow (Gronthos et al., 1994), whereas negative in human adipose-derived MSCs (AD-MSCs) (Gronthos, et al., 20019),

4.4. Clinical Application of MSCs in DFUs

There is a need to develop novel therapies for treatment of non-healing diabetic ulcers in order to prevent amputation and reduce the significant financial burden on individual and society. The understanding of the pathophysiology of diabetic wound healing is important for the development of advanced wound healing treatments. It allows therapeutic targeting of the different phases of wound healing. For the isolation of MSCs, bone marrow is one of the most common tissues. BM-MSCs have no immunologic restriction and do not stimulate alloreactivity because they have capability of escaping lysis by cytotoxic T-cell and natural killer (NK) cells (Le Blanc, 2003). Autologous stem cell was administered to the patients with DFUs, our analysis suggests that stem cell treatment is safe and significantly helps diabetic ulcer healing (Dash et al., 2009: 2014), without any increased risk of treatment-related adverse events. The most frequently used MSCs are BM-MSC, PB-MSC, hUC-MSC. Kim et al. (2012) reported enhanced wound healing with secretion of angiogenic factors and enhanced engraftment/differentiation capabilities with the use of intradermal injections of human amniotic MSC in a diabetic mouse wound model. Similarly, Zheng et al. (2017) showed that improved ulcer healing in diabetic mice with topical application of micronized amniotic membrane containing human amniotic epithelial cells compared to decellularized membrane. Kong et al. (2013) reported wound healing with intradermal injection of human placental MSC in diabetic Goto-Kakizaki rats. Locally applied MSC are sufficient to enhanced wound healing after injection of collagen gels containing embryonic fetal liver MSC in diabetic Lep *db/db* mice compared to CD45+ cell treatment (Badillo et al. 2007). Barcelos et al. (2009) used a collagen hydrogel scaffold to deliver human fetal aortic MSC in a murine DFU model. Use of MSCs in regenerative and reparative therapies for neurological disorders are reported (Khoo et al., 2011). BM- MSCs and other sources of MSCs have been explored actively in recent years, but their biology remains poorly understood. BM-MSCs are easy to isolate, expand, characterize, and differentiate into many cell lineages. Hence most of the current research focus on MSC application are centered on BM-MSCs. BM-MSCs constitute nearly 10% of the hematopoietic stem cells (HSCs), and they are always regarded as a component of the HSC niche (Friedenstein et al., 1966). Autologous BM-MSCs have shown efficacy for the treatment of the non-healing diabetic ulcers (Dash et al., 2009). Vojtassak et al. (2006) used autologous biograft composed of autologous skin fibroblasts on biodegradable collagen membrane (Coladerm) combined with autologous mesenchymal stem cells (MSC) derived from the patient's bone marrow. There was overall decreased in wound size and an increase in the vascularity of the dermis and in the dermal thickness of the wound bed after 29 days of combined treatment. BM- MSCs participate in all phases of wound healing and help to reconstitute the dermal, vascular, and other components required for optimal healing (Al-Khalidi et al., 2003). Critical limb ischaemia DFU patients transplanted with bone marrow mononuclear cells (BMCs) and expanded bone marrow cells enriched in CD90+ cells ('tissue repair cells', TRCs), and the study proved that transplantation of BMCs as well as TRCs proved to be safe and feasible. Improvements of microcirculation and complete wound healing were observed in the transplant groups (Kirana et al., 2012).

4.5. Mechanism of Action of MSCs in DFUs

A comprehensive understanding of the mechanism of action is required to apprehend the therapeutic potential of MSCs. MSCs can be evaluated by its ability to differentiate and transdifferentiate into tissue-specific cells, to fuse with the resident cells, and secretion of paracrine factors in order to regulate the local microenvironment and immune response. The possible therapeutic mechanisms behind MSCs action for healing DFUs may be-

Table 2. Clinical trials for DFUs using autologous MSCs

Type of cells administrated	Route of administration	Outcome from the experiment	Follow up period (months)	Reference
Autologous PBMNCs	Subcutaneous injections and intra-mascular	Limb ulcers (77.8%) of patients were completely healed	3	Huang et al., 2005
Autologous BM-MCS	Intra-muscular and subcutaneous	The ulcer healing, rest pain and intermittent claudication were improved significantly.	3	Debin et al., 2008
Autologous BM-MCS	Intra-muscular	Blood stream of lower limbs increased	3	Chen B et al., 2009
Autologous BM-MCS	Intra-muscular	Development of dermal cells, nonhealing ulcers accelerates the healing process and improves clinical parameters significantly	3	Dash et al., 2009
Autologous BM-MCS	Intra-muscular	BMMSCs therapy may be better tolerated and more effective than BMMNCs for increasing lower limb perfusion and promoting foot ulcer healing in diabetic patients with CLI (critical limb ischemia).	6	Lu et al. 2011
Autologous BM-MCS	Injection and spray	BM-MSC showed better ulcer healing	3	Jain et al., 2011
Autologous BM-MCS	Intra-mascular and intra-arterial	Improvements of microcirculation and complete wound healing were observed in the transplant groups.	11	Kirana et al. 2012
Autologous PB-MCS	Intra-muscular	Angiogenesis and improvement in the healing process in diabetic patients with CLI	3	Mohammadzadeh et al., 2013
Autologous PB-MCS	Intra-arterial and intra-muscular	Promotes the establishment of collateral circulation in patients with diabetic foot, improvement of life quality, pain, cold sensation, clinical symptoms and ulcer healing	15	XU et al., 2016
Allogeneic hUC-MSC	Intra-arterial and intra-muscular	Significant increase in neovessels, accompanied by complete or gradual ulcer healing.	3	Qin et al., 2016

4.5.1. Anti-Inflammatory Action

MSCs influence the wound's ability to progress beyond the inflammatory phase and not regress to a chronic wound state. MSCs inhibit macrophage pro-inflammatory cytokine production, such as tumor necrosis factor-a (TNF-a), IL- 6, and interferon-a (IFN-a37 and stimulate anti-inflammatory cytokine IL-10 and IL-12 production (Ne´meth et al., 2009). By doing so, immune cell activation and local inflammatory processes are limited, reducing tissue damage. Cytokine secretion by MSCs has an influence on immune system and other cells responsible for wound healing. Post-injury T cells secrete pro-inflammatory cytokines, which may stall the wound in inflammatory phase. MSCs can suppress several T lymphocyte activities both *in vitro* and *in vivo* by secreting mediators such as IL-10, transforming growth factor-b (TGF-b), indoleamine 2,3-dioxygenase (IDO), nitric oxide (NO), and prostaglandin E2 (PGE2) (Ren et al., 2008). IDO induces the depletion of tryptophan from the local environment, which is essential for lymphocyte proliferation. NO mediates its effect partly through phosphorylation of signal transducer and activator of transcription-5 (STAT-5), which results in suppression of T cell proliferation, by inhibiting either NO synthase or prostaglandin synthesis. In addition to its effect on the Janus kinase (JAK)/STAT pathway, NO may also influence mitogen-activated protein kinase (MAPK) and nuclear factor-jB (NF-jB), which reduces the gene expression of pro-inflammatory cytokines. MSCs can suppress the activation of M1 macrophages (pro-inflammatory form) and induce proliferation of M2 macrophages (anti-inflammatory form), thereby favoring secretion of anti-inflammatory cytokines, and enhance resolution of chronic inflammation.

MSCs inhibit neutrophil migration and decrease their ROS production, but at the same time do not decrease their phagocytic capacity. MSCs also assist in clearing the wound site by promoting apoptotic cell phagocytosis. These anti-inflammatory properties of MSCs make them beneficial to the healing process of chronic ulcers because they force the stalled wound to advance past a chronic inflammatory state into the next stage of healing.

4.5.2. Role in Angiogenesis

Angiogenic support provided by MSCs is vital for recovery of damaged tissues. MSCs secrete SDF-1, VEGF, and other cytokines important for angiogenesis like basic fibroblast growth factor (bFGF) and MMPs. SDF-1 activity is essential for endothelial cell survival, vascular branching, and pericyte recruitment (Yamhguchi et al., 2003). VEGF, apart from being a potent angiogenic cytokine, not only mobilizes EPCs from bone marrow but also inhibits EPC apoptosis. In the proliferative stage, MSCs reinforce vascular supply by secreting a number of angiogenic factors and facilitate production of ECM. BM-MSCs in diabetic wounds also improved collagen levels (types I–V) in the wound bed. (Kwon et al., 2008).

4.5.3. Paracrine Secretion of Growth Factors and Cytokines

The paracrine action includes secretion of cytokines, growth factors, and chemokines that regulate a number of cells, such as epithelial cells, endothelial cells, keratinocytes, and fibroblasts, and has productive effects on immunoregulation, angiogenesis, epithelialization, and fibroproliferation during wound repair. Analysis of paracrine factors released by BM-MSCs shows that BM-MSCs secreted distinctively increased amounts of VEGF-α, insulin-like growth factor-1 (IGF-1), epidermal growth factor (EGF), keratinocyte growth factor, angiopoietin-1, stromal cell–derived factor-1 (SDF-1), macrophage inflammatory protein-1a and -b, and erythropoietin. These molecules are known to be important in normal wound healing (Chen et al., 2008). MSCs secrete a variety of cytokines and growth factors that have anti-fibrotic properties, including hepatic growth factor (HGF), IL-10, adrenomedullin, (Li et al., 2008) and MMP-9, (Kim et al., 2011) that promote turnover of the ECM, (Schievenbusch et al., 2009) keratinocyte proliferation, (Bevan et al., 2004) and inhibition of myofibroblast differentiation (Shukla et al., 2009).

4.5.4. Direct Differentiation into Skin Components

MSCs have been shown to differentiate into cardiomyocytes, adipocytes, chondrocytes, neuronal cells, and dermal epithelial cells. *In vivo* and *in vitro*, it has been shown that MSCs can differentiate into epidermal keratinocytes and other skin appendages. In a wound environment, MSC differentiate into keratinocytes and express keratinocyte-specific keratin protein (Wu et al., 2007).

5. Limitation with Current Cell Based Therapy

Autologous BM-MSCs shows efficacy in cell therapy for DFU patients. Most recently, a study on the feasibility of autologous stem cell therapy in diabetic patients showed that adipose tissue-derived mesenchymal stem cells isolated from distal limbs of diabetic patients with critical ischemia was not reasonable (Koc et al., 2014), the study concluded that reduced expression of VEGF (vascular endothelial growth factor) as well as reduced osteogenic differentiation may have an impact on the effectiveness of autologous cell therapies in diabetic patients. A comprehensive understanding of the immunological profile is essential for autologous or allogeneic MSCs to be used in improving diabetic wound healing studies. Allogeneic MSCs have potent immunosuppressive properties, evidence also suggests that they can be a potential new therapeutic strategy for the treatment of DFU in animal models. Allogeneic UCB-MSCs have been successfully used to treat patients with DFU (Pane's et al., 2016).

Methodological flaws in the clinical trials have raised concerns over the validity of the results and that is most important reason for creating a barrier in treatment of DFUs. Systematic reviews have been reported on statistical benefit in wound healing. However, there is lack of information on safety, method of recruitment, randomization methods and blinding strategy for outcome assessments. Another flaw is lack of power size calculations in some of the trials and little mention of dropouts in trial. However, the lack of clinical success with advanced products is not solely due to the aforementioned flaws in trial design. There are several limitations in the reported studies. Stem cell sources, the number of delivered cells, and the routes of cell administration differed among the studies. Due to these significant heterogeneities, optimized procedure protocols were not determined. To explore the feasibility of autologous and allogeneic MSCs therapy in DFU a large number of preclinical and clinical data required.

MSCs are the most commonly used stem cells in current clinical applications. Although significant progress has been made in stem cell research in recent years, cell therapy with stem cells is far from a mature clinical technology. MSCs are considered for therapy because they are free from ethical issues and available from numerous sources, low immunogenicity and no teratoma risk however, there are still several major hurdles to their widespread utility. It is still not known which source should be used for which disease, and the route of administration best suited for a particular disease, and possible contraindications to their clinical use. Once administered, the parameters for monitoring clinical effectiveness also need to be established and are likely to vary for different disorders. Most importantly, established standards for cell expansion protocols, product quality, and safety controls are not available in most countries. Furthermore, studies on interactions between MSCs and the inflammatory milieu in which they reside, and the therapeutic mechanisms are still lacking. The large-scale application of MSCs is a newly emerging and rapidly advancing field but benefited patients suffer a wide array of side effects. Government regulatory agencies are eagerly waiting for detailed answers to these questions for the establishment of a regulatory polices to meet the challenges. Future use of soluble products of MSCs instead of MSCs themselves with proper screening, may simplify the administration and make it safer.

6. FUTURE DIRECTIONS

Future directions for MSC transplantations in chronic wound contexts might focus on optimization of delivery systems as well as improving cell survival via independent technologies or in combination with these delivery systems. MSCs adaptability in the new environment has made them a potential tool for disease treatment, though the full understanding of MSCs mechanism is still in their preliminary stages. Some promising technologies outlined in several clinical trials are basic fibrin mesh scaffolds in gel form for seeding of MSCs. Recent breakthrough discoveries in BM-MSCs delivered by this EGF microspheres-based engineered skin model have made it an ideal source for future cell therapy in regenerative medicine (Huang et al., 2012). Recent studies showed that a transgenic *L. sericata* larvae could secrete platelet derived growth factor-BB (PDGF-BB), a dimeric peptide growth factor that could bind to the platelet derived growth factor (PDGF) receptor and stimulate cell proliferation and survival, and, hence, promote wound healing (Linger et al., 2016). It may be cost-effective for DFUs and can be employed in regenerative medicine. Studies on immunomodulation of MSCs and wound support in other wound models (myocardial infarction, brain, long bone defects, and others) may support progressive wound care research in cell therapy.

The clinician must be aware that the majority of biological products are composed of high levels of proteins. Proteins may be very sensitive to inflammatory enzymatic activity in a wound. Controlling high levels of inflammation is as critical as debridement in promoting wound healing. When choosing any biological or advanced modality, it is essential that the clinician compares average time to complete closure provided by well-designed randomized controlled studies with healing time provided by less-expensive standard approaches to wound care. Often, the time to healing with expensive and advanced modalities is not significantly different to that from inexpensive standard approaches to treatment of the diabetic ulcer. Regardless of the product used, off-loading the diabetic foot is critical to successful wound closure. Even the most advanced product may fail in the presence of repetitive trauma and pressure. Technologies for various molecular analyses (such as genomics, proteomics, systems for sustained topical delivery (such as polymers and adenovirus vectors), major advances in tissue engineering (such as human skin engineering, cellular matrices, and bone marrow–derived cell therapy), novel discoveries of disease molecular pathogenesis from studies of patient biopsies and animal models, coupled with breakthroughs in stem cell research, hold the promise of a bright future.

CONCLUSION

In conclusion, several reports suggest that the autologous mesenchymal stem cell-based therapy is efficient and safe for the treatment of lower extremity ulcer caused by ischemia or diabetes. Cell therapies for improving wound healing have become a topic of great interest, particularly for non-healing wounds such as diabetic foot. Despite some potential limitations, we have here outlined several reasons how mesenchymal stem cells provide unique and effective support for stimulating the wound healing process in a chronic wound bed including its ability to suppress excessive inflammation while stimulating *de novo* angiogenesis in the wound bed leading to promising outcomes in chronic wound repair.

ACKNOWLEDGMENTS

This work was supported by SCB Medical College Cuttack, Odisha, India from an internal funding of the Institute.

REFERENCES

Al-Khalidi, A., Al-Sabiti, H., Galipeau, J. & Lachapelle, K. (2003). Therapeutic angiogenesis using autologous bone marrow stromal cells improved blood flow in chronic limb ischemia model. *Ann. Thoracic Surg.*, 75, 204–209.

Allickson, J. G., Sanchez, A., Yefimenko, N., Borlongan, C. V. & Sanberg, P. R. (2011). Recent studies assessing the proliferative capability of a novel adult stem cell identified in menstrual blood. *Open Stem Cell J.*, *3*, 4–10.

American Diabetes Association (2009). Diagnosis and classification of diabetes mellitus. *Diab care.*, (2009), *32*, (Suppl 1), S62–S67. https://doi.org/10.2337/dc09-S062.

Armstrong, D. G., Wrobe, J. & Robbins, J. M. (2007). Guest editorial: are diabetes-related wounds and amputations worse than cancer? *Int Wound J.*, *4*, 286–287.

Badillo, A. T., Redden, R. A., Zhang, L., Doolin, E. J. & Liechty, K. W. (2007). Treatment of diabetic wounds with fetal murine mesenchymal stromal cells enhances wound closure. *Cell Tissue Res.*, *329*, 301-311.

Barcelos, L. S., Duplaa, C., Krankel, N., Graiani, G., Invernici, G., Katare, R., Siragusa, M., Meloni, M., Campesi, I., Monica, M., Simm, A., Campagnolo, P., Mangialardi, G., Stevanato, L., Alessandri, G., Emanueli, C. & Madeddu, P. (2009). Human CD133+ progenitor cells promote the healing of diabetic ischemic ulcers by paracrine stimulation of angiogenesis and activation of Wnt signaling. *Circ. Res.*, *104*, 1095–1102.

Bourne, R. R., Stevens, G. A., White, R. A., Smith, J. L., Flaxman, S. R., Price, H., Jonas, J. B., Keeffe, J., Leasher, J., Naidu, K., Pseudovas, K., Resinkoff, S. & Taylor H. R. (2013). Causes of vision loss worldwide, 1990–2010: a systematic analysis. *Lancet Global Health.*, *1*, (6), e339-e349.

Dash, N. R., Dash, S. N., Routray, P., Mohapatra, S. & Mohapatra, P. C. (2009). Targeting nonhealing ulcers of lower extremity in human through autologous bone marrow-derived mesenchymal stem cells. *Rejuvenation Res.*, *12*(5), 359-366.

Dash, S. N., Dash, N. R., Guru, B. & Mohapatra, P. C. (2014). Towards reaching the target: clinical application of mesenchymal stem cells for diabetic foot ulcers. *Rejuvenation Res.*, *17*(1), 40-53.

Dreifke, M. B., Jayasuriya, A. A. & Jayasuriya, A. C. (2015). Current wound healing procedures and potential care. *Mater Sci Eng C Materl Biol Appl.*, *48*, 651-662.

Friedenstein, A. J., Piatetzky-Shapiro, I. & Petrakova, K. V. (1966). Osteogenesis in transplants of bone marrow cells. *J Embryol Exp Morph*, *16*, 381–390.

Frykberg, R. G., Zgonis, T., Armstrong, D. G., Driver, V. R., Giurini, J. M., Kravitz, S. R., Landsman, A. S., Lavery, L. A., Moore, J. C., Schuberth, J. M., Wukich, D. K., Andersen, C. & Vanore, J. V. (2006). American College of Foot and Ankle Surgeons. Diabetic foot disorders. A clinical practice guideline (2006 revision). *J Foot Ankle Surg.*, *45*, (5 Suppl), S1-66.

Gronthos, S., Franklin, D. M., Leddy, H. A., Robey, P. G., Storms, R. W. & Gimble, J. M. (2001). Surface protein characterization of human adipose tissue-derived stromal cells. *J. Cell Physiol.*, *189*, 54–63.

Gronthos, S., Graves, S. E., Ohta, S. & Simmons, P. J. (1994). The STRO-1 + fraction of adult human bone marrow contains the osteogenic precursors. *Blood*, *84*, 4164–4173.

Horwitz, E. M., Le Blanc, K., Dominici, M., Mueller, I., Slaper-Cortenbach, I., Marini, F. C., Deans, R. J., Krause, D. S. & Keating, A. (2005). International Society for Cellular Therapy. Clarification of the nomenclature for MSC: The International Society for Cellular Therapy position statement. *Cytotherapy*, *7*, 393–395.

Huang, S., Lu, G., Wu, Y., Jirigala, E., Xu, Y., Ma, K. & Fu, X. (2012). Mesenchymal stem cells delivered in a microsphere-based engineered skin contribute to cutaneous wound healing and sweat gland repair. *J Dermatol Sci.*, *66*(1), 29-36.

In't Anker, P. S., Scherjon, S. A., Kleijburg-vander Keur, C., Noort, W. A., Claas, F. H., Willemze, R., Fibbe, W. E. & Kanhai, H. H. (2003) Amniotic fluid as a novel source of mesenchymal stem cells for therapeutic transplantation. *Blood*, *102*, 1548–1549.

Jiao, F., Wang, J., Dong, Z. L., Wu, M. J., Zhao, T. B., Li, D. D. & Wang, X. (2012). Human mesenchymal stem cells derived from limb bud can differentiate into all three embryonic germ layers lineages. *Cell Reprogram.*, *14*, 324–333.

Kadar, K., Kiraly, M., Porcsalmy, B., Molnar, B., Racz, G. Z., Blazsek, J., Kallo, K., Szabo, E. L., Gera, I., Gerber, G. & Varga, G. (2009).

Differentiation potential of stem cells from human dental origin - promise for tissue engineering. *J. Physiol. Pharmacol.*, 60 (7), 167–175.

Kadir, Ab. R., Zainal Ariffin, S. H., Megat, Abdul Wahab, R., Kermani, S. & Senafi, S. (2012). Characterization of mononucleated human peripheral blood cells. *Scientific World Journal*, 2012, 843843.

Khoo, M. L. M., Tao, H. & Ma, D. D. F. (2011). Mesenchymal stem cell-based therapies for Parkinson's disease: Progress, controversies and lessons for the future. *J Stem Cell Res Ther.*, 2011, S2, 005.

Kim, C. H., Lee, J. H., Won, J. H. & Cho, M. K. (2011). Mesenchymal stem cells improve wound healing *in vivo* via early activation of matrix metalloproteinase-9 and vascular endothelial growth factor. *J Korean Med Sci.*, 26, 726–733.

Kim, S. W., Zhang, H. Z., Guo, L., Kim, J. M. & Kim, M. H. (2012). Amniotic mesenchymal stem cells enhance wound healing in diabetic NOD/SCID mice through high angiogenic and engraftment capabilities. *PLoS One*, 7, e41105.

Kirana, S., Stratmann, B., Prante, C., Prohaska, W., Koerperich, H., Lammers, D., Gastens, M. H., Quast, T., Negrean, M., Stirban, O. A., Nandrean, S. G., Gotting, C., Minartz, P., Kleesiek, K. & Tschoepe, D. (2012). Autologous stem cell therapy in the treatment of limb ischaemia induced chronic tissue ulcers of diabetic foot patients. *Int J Clin Pract.*, 66, 384–93.

Kočí, Z., Turnovcová, K., Dubský, M., Baranovičová, L., Holáň, V., Chudíčková, M., Syková, E. & Kubinová, S. (2014). Characterization of human adipose tissue-derived stromal cells isolated from diabetic patient's distal limbs with critical ischemia. *Cell Bio- chemistry and Function*, 32, 597–604.

Kong, P., Xie, X., Li, F., Liu, Y. & Lu, Y. (2013). Placenta mesenchymal stem cell accelerates wound healing by enhancing angiogenesis in diabetic Goto-Kakizaki (GK) rats. *Biochem Biophys Res Commun.*, 438, 410–9.

Kwon, D. S., Gao, X., Liu, Y. B., Dulchavsky, D. S., Danyluk, A. L., Bansal, M., Chopp, M., McIntosh, K., Arbab, A. S., Dulchavsky, S. A.

& Gautam, S. C. (2008). Treatment with bone marrow-derived stromal cells accelerates wound healing in diabetic rats. *Int. Wound J.*, *5*, 453–463.

Le Blanc, K. (2003). Immunomodulatory effects of fetal and adult mesenchymal stem cells. *Cytotherapy*, 5(6). 485–489, 2003.

Li, L., Zhang, Y., Li, Y., Yu, B., Xu, Y., Zhao, S. & Guan, Z. (2008) Mesenchymal stem cell transplantation attenuates cardiac fibrosis associated with isoproterenol-induced global heart failure. *Transpl Int.*, *21*, 1181–1189.

Lin, C. S., Ning, H., Lin, G. & Lue, T. F. (2012). Is CD34 truly a negative marker for mesenchymal stromal cells? *Cytotherapy*, *14*, 1159–1163.

Linger, R. J., Belikoff, E. J., Yan, Y., Li, F., Wantuch, H. A., Fitzsimons, H. L. & Scott, M. J. (2016). Towards next generation maggot debridement therapy: transgenic *Lucilia sericata* larvae that produce and secrete a human growth factor. *BMC Biotechnol.*, *22*, 16-30.

Margolis, D. J., Malay, D. S., Hoffstad, O, J., Leonard, C, E., Thomas MaCurdy, T., Tan, Y., Molina, T., López de Nava, K. & Siegel, K. (2013). Economic burden of diabetic foot ulcers and amputations. Data Points #3; Data Points Publication Series [Internet], 2008. Accessed 12 August 2013; https://www.ncbi.nlm.nih.gov/ books/NBK 65152/pdf/Bookshelf_NBK65152.pdf.

Morito, T., Muneta, T., Hara, K., Ju, Y. J., Mochizuki, T., Makino, H., Umezawa, A. & Sekiya, I. (2008). Synovial fluid-derived mesenchymal stem cells increase after intra-articular ligament injury in humans. *Rheumatology*, *47*, 1137–1143.

Moxey, P. W., Gogalniceanu, P., Hinchliffe, R. J., Loftus, I. M., Jones, K. J. & Thompson, M. M. (2011). Lower extremity amputations – a review of global variability in incidence. *Diabetic Medicine*, *28* (10), 1144–1153.

Ne´meth, K., Leelahavanichkul, A., Yuen, P. S., Mayer, B., Parmelee, A., Doi, K., Robey, P. G., Leelahavanichkul, K., Koller, B. H., Brown, J. M., Hu, X., Jelinek, I., Star, R. A. & Mezey, E. (2009). Bone marrow stromal cells attenuate sepsis via prostaglandin E (2)-dependent reprogramming of host macrophages to increase their interleukin-10 production. *Nat Medicine, 15*, 42–49.

Panés, J., García-Olmo, D., Van Assche, G., Colombel, J. F., Reinisch, W., Baumgart, D. C., Dignass, A., Nachury, M., Ferrante, M., Kazemi-Shirazi, L., Grimaud, J. C., de la Portilla, F., Goldin, E., Richard, M. P., Leselbaum, A. & Danese, S. (2016). ADMIRE CD Study Group Collaborators. Expanded allogeneic adipose-derived mesenchymal stem cells (Cx601) for complex perianal fistulas in Crohn's disease: a phase 3 randomized, double-blind controlled trial," *The Lancet, 388*, 1281–1290.

Park, B. W., Kang, D. H., Kang, E. J., Byun, J. H., Lee, J. S., Maeng, G. H. & Rho, G. J. (2012). Peripheral nerve regeneration using autologous porcine skin-derived mesenchymal stem cells. *J Tissue Eng Regen Med., 6*(2), 113-24.

Park, J. C., Kim, J. M., Jung, I. H., Kim, J. C., Choi, S. H., Cho, K. S. & Kim, C. S. (2011). Isolation and characterization of human periodontal ligament (PDL) stem cells (PDLSCs) from the inflamed PDL tissue: *in vitro* and *in vivo* evaluations. *J. Clin. Periodontol., 38*, 721–731.

Pecoraro, R. E., Reiber, G. E. & Burgess, E. M. (1990). Pathways to diabetic limb amputation. Basis for prevention. *Diabetes Care, 13*, 513–521.

Pittenger, M. F., Mackay, A. M., Beck, S. C., Jaiswal, R. K., Douglas, R., Mosca, J. D., Moorman, M. A., Simonetti, D. W., Craig, S. & Marshak, D. R. (1999). Multilineage potential of adult human mesenchymal stem cells. *Science, 284*, 143–147.

Raynaud, C. M., Maleki, M., Lis, R., Ahmed, B., Al-Azwani, I., Malek, J., Safadi, F. F. & Rafii, A. (2012). Comprehensive characterization of mesenchymal stem cells from human placenta and fetal membrane and their response to osteoactivin stimulation. *Stem Cells Int., 2012*, 658356.

Ren, G., Zhang, L., Zhao, X., Xu, G., Zhang, Y., Roberts, A. I., Zhao, R. C. & Shi, Y. (2008). Mesenchymal stem cell-mediated immunosuppression occurs via concerted action of chemokines and nitric oxide. *Cell Stem Cell, 2*, 141–150.

Sarwar, N., Gao, P., Seshasai, S. R., Gobin, R., Kaptoge, S., Di Angelantonio, E., Ingelsson, E., Lawlor, D. A., Selvin, E., Stampfer, M., Stehouwer, C. D., Lewington, S., Pennells, L., Thompson, A., Sattar, N., White, I. R., Ray, K. K. & Danesh, J. (2010). Diabetes mellitus, fasting blood glucose concentration, and risk of vascular disease: a collaborative meta-analysis of 102 prospective studies. Emerging Risk Factors Collaboration. *Lancet.*, *26*, 375, 2215-2222.

Schievenbusch, S., Strack, I., Scheffler, M., Wennhold, K., Maurer, J., Nischt, R., Dienes, H. P. & Odenthal, M. (2009). Profiling of anti-fibrotic signaling by hepatocyte growth factor in renal fibroblasts. *Biochem Biophys Res Commun.*, *385*, 55–61.

Schuring, A. N., Schulte, N., Kelsch, R., Ropke, A., Kiesel, L. & Gotte, M. (2011). Characterization of endometrial mesenchymal stem-like cells obtained by endometrial biopsy during routine diagnostics. *Fertil. Steril.*, *95*, 423–426.

Shukla, M. N., Rose, J. L., Ray, R., Lathrop, K. L., Ray, A. & Ray, P. (2009). Hepatocyte growth factor inhibits epithelial to myofibroblast transition in lung cells via Smad7. *Am J Respir Cell Mol Biol.*, *40*, 643–653.

Tsai, M. S., Lee, J. L., Chang, Y. J. & Hwang, S. M. (2004). Isolation of human multipotent mesenchymal stem cells from second-trimester amniotic fluid using a novel two-stage culture protocol. *Hum. Reprod.*, *19*, 1450–1456.

Vaculik, C., Schuster, C., Bauer, W., Iram, N., Pfisterer, K., Kramer, G., Reinisch, A., Strunk, D. & Elbe-Burger, A. (2012). Human dermis harbors distinct mesenchymal stromal cell subsets. *J. Invest. Dermatol.*, *132*, (3 Pt 1), 563–574.

Vojtassak, J., Danisovic, L., Kubes, M., Bakos, D., Jarabek, L., Ulicna, M. & Blasko, M. (2006). Autologous biograft and mesenchymal stem cells in treatment of the diabetic foot. *Neuro Endocrinol Lett.*, *27*, (Suppl. 2), 134–137.

Wagner, W., Wein, F., Seckinger, A., Frankhauser, M., Wirkner, U., Krause, U., Blake, J., Schwager, C., Eckstein, V., Ansorge, W. & Ho, A. D. (2005). Comparative characteristics of mesenchymal stem cells from human bone marrow, adipose tissue, and umbilical cord blood. *Exp. Hematol.*, *33*, 1402–1416.

Wang, H. S., Hung, S. C., Peng, S. T. & Chen, C. C. (2004). Mesenchymal stem cells in the Wharton's jelly of the human umbilical cord. *Stem Cells*, *22*, 330–1337.

Wei, X., Yang, X., Han, Z. P., Qu, F. F., Shao, L. & Shi, Y. F. (2013). Mesenchymal stem cells: a new trend for cell therapy. *Acta Pharmacol. Sin.*, *34*, 747–754.

World Health Organization (1999). *Definition, diagnosis and classification of diabetes mellitus and its complications. Part 1: Diagnosis and classification of diabetes mellitus.* WHO/NCD/NCS/99.2. Geneva: World Health Organization. Retrieved from: https://apps.who.int/iris/handle/10665/66040.

Wu, Y., Chen, L., Scott, P. G. & Tredget, E. E. (2007). Mesenchymal stem cells enhance wound healing through differentiation and angiogenesis. *Stem Cells.*, *25*, 2648–2659.

Yamaguchi, J., Kusano, K. F., Masuo, O., Kawamoto, A., Silver, M., Murasawa, S., Bosch-Marce, M., Masuda, H., Losordo, D. W., Isner, J. M. & Asahara, T. (2003). Stromal cell-derived factor-1 effect on ex vivo expanded endothelial progenitor cell recruitment for ischemic neovascularization. *Circulation*, *107*, 1322–1328.

Zhang, X., Hirai, M., Cantero, S., Ciubotariu, R., Dobrila, L., Hirsh, A., Igura, K., Satoh, H., Yokomi, I., Nishimura, T., Yamaguchi, S., Yoshimura, K., Rubinstein, P. & Takahashi, T. A. (2011). Isolation and characterization of mesenchymal stem cells from human umbilical cord blood: reevaluation of critical factors for successful isolation and high ability to proliferate and differentiate to chondrocytes as compared to mesenchymal stem cells from bone marrow and adipose tissue. *J Cell Biochem.*, *112*(4), 1206-1218.

Zheng, Y., Ji, S., Wu, H., Tian, S., Zhang, Y., Wang, L., Fang, H., Luo, P., Wang, X., Hu, X., Xiao, S. & Xia, Z. (2017). Topical administration of cryopreserved living micronized amnion accelerates wound healing in diabetic mice by modulating local microenvironment. *Biomaterials.*, *113*, 56–67.

In: Diabetic Foot: Prevention and Treatment ISBN: 978-1-53616-266-0
Editor: Gianni Romano © 2019 Nova Science Publishers, Inc.

Chapter 3

ARE ANTIMICROBIAL PEPTIDES THE ANSWER FOR DIABETIC FOOT INFECTION MANAGEMENT?

Raquel Santos[1,2], *Luís Tavares*[1] *and Manuela Oliveira*[1,*]

[1]CIISA-Centro de Investigação Interdisciplinar em Sanidade Animal, Faculdade de Medicina Veterinária, Universidade de Lisboa, Lisboa, Portugal
[2]Instituto de Medicina Molecular, Faculdade de Medicina, Universidade de Lisboa, Lisboa, Portugal

ABSTRACT

Diabetes *mellitus* is a serious health problem that has shown an increasing prevalence in the last decades, affecting more than 422 million people globally nowadays. As a consequence of multiple pathophysiological factors, namely neuropathy, vasculopathy and immunopathy, the lifetime risk for diabetic patients of developing a foot ulcer can be as high as 25%. Approximately half of these ulcers can become clinically infected, usually by opportunistic pathogens, including

---

[*] Corresponding Author's E-mail: moliveira@fmv.ulisboa.pt.

both aerobic and anaerobic bacteria and yeasts. Due to local microenvironmental conditions unfavorable to wound healing, infected ulcers may result in purulent discharge, intense inflammation and progressive tissue damage.

Several bacteria are related with diabetic foot infections (DFIs), mainly *Staphylococcus* spp., *Enterococcus* spp., *Streptococcus* spp., *Enterobacteriaceae*, *Pseudomonas* spp., *Acinetobacter* spp. and *Peptoniphilus* spp. These species have the ability to express numerous virulence factors that are putatively involved in their pathogenicity, including quorum-sensing molecules and biofilm structures. Moreover, DFI pathogens are known for their antibiotic resistance profile. The increasing prevalence of multidrug resistant isolates, formation of biofilms and inadequate wound healing found in DFIs may impair the successful outcome of conventional anti-infectious therapeutics in these patients. In fact, foot gangrene subsequent to a non-healing DFI is nowadays the leading cause of non-traumatic lower limb amputations.

Antimicrobial peptides (AMPs) have emerged as a potential strategy to be used in combination with or as an alternative to conventional antibiotherapy in the management of chronic DFIs. AMPs are amphipathic molecules containing cationic and hydrophobic amino acid residues, enabling them to form non-specific interactions with the negatively charged bacterial membranes. There are several studies available regarding the activity of these small peptides, providing information on their antimicrobial spectrum, mechanisms of action and biological effects in wound healing.

Nisin and pexiganan are two of the most promising AMPs for application against antibiotic resistant bacteria. Both nisin and pexiganan are able to disrupt prokaryotic membranes, inducing a fast killing of bacteria. Nisin binds to the peptidoglycan precursor lipid II, inhibiting cell wall synthesis and promoting pore formation on bacterial cytoplasmic membranes; on the other hand, pexiganan exerts its antibacterial effect via toroidal pore formation. The multiple mechanisms of action, the quick onset of activity and the low specificity in terms of molecular targets decreases the tendency of bacteria to develop resistance towards AMPs.

Given the increasing prevalence of antibiotic resistant pathogens and, consequently, the failure of antibiotic-exclusive therapeutics in DFIs treatment, combinations involving AMPs and antibiotics may be a potential treatment alternative in a near future.

Keywords: antimicrobial peptides, diabetic foot infection, nisin, pexiganan

DIABETIC FOOT INFECTION

Diabetes *mellitus* is a chronic disease that affects more than 422 million people worldwide and which prevalence is expected to double by 2030 (World Health Organization 2016). Diabetic patients have a predisposition to develop vascular, neurological and immunological diseases, being peripheral neuropathy and lower extremity arterial disease the main factors responsible for the onset of diabetic foot ulceration (Armstrong, et al. 2011). Secondary to multiple pathophysiological factors, including diabetes-associated immunopathy, diabetic patients are unable to establish a normal inflammatory response against microbial pathogens, and diabetic foot infection (DFI) following ulceration of the protective skin is a common and devastating complication presented by these patients (Hobizal and Wukich 2012).

Diabetic foot ulcers (DFUs) represent one of the most severe complications of diabetes, affecting up to a quarter of diabetic patients, being expected that during their lifetime, approximately half of these ulcers will become clinically infected (Hobizal and Wukich 2012).

Although ischemic and neuropathic lesions promote the DFU onset, it is the infection by pathogenic microorganisms along with the local microenvironmental conditions unfavorable to antibiotics action that are ultimately responsible for DFI recalcitrance (Armstrong, et al. 2011, Lipsky, Aragón-Sánchez, et al. 2016). Chronically infected DFUs, characterized by severe inflammation and progressive tissue damage with the involvement of bacterial biofilms, are often resistant to antibiotherapy and can evolve to gangrene. As a result, DFIs are the most common diabetic complications requiring hospitalization and the worldwide leading cause of non-traumatic lower extremity amputation (Lipsky, Aragón-Sánchez, et al. 2016). In fact, it is estimated that more than 60% of non-traumatic lower limb amputations occur in diabetic patients (Kosinski and Lipsky 2010, Yazdanpanah, Nasiri and Adarvishi 2015), with these patients presenting a lower limb amputation rate of 15 times higher than patients without diabetes (Yazdanpanah, Nasiri and Adarvishi 2015).

ASSOCIATED MICROBIOTA

Diabetes-associated foot infections are caused by a polymicrobial community of pathogens. While Gram-positive bacteria, including *Staphylococcus* spp., *Streptococcus* spp., *Enterococcus* spp. and *Corynebacterium* spp. tend to predominate in acute DFIs, the microbiota of chronic DFIs is mainly constituted by Gram-negative bacteria, such as *Pseudomonas* spp., *Proteus* spp., *Acinetobacter* spp. and *Klebsiella* spp., followed by anaerobes, namely *Peptoniphilus* spp. and *Bacteroides* spp. (Lipsky, Berendt, et al. 2012, Mendes, et al. 2012, Banu, et al. 2015). Despite the variety of pathogens associated to DFIs, epidemiological studies report a clear predominance of *Staphylococcus aureus* and *Pseudomonas aeruginosa* as the main Gram-positive and Gram-negative bacteria, respectively, present in these infections (Mendes, et al. 2012, Banu, et al. 2015).

The microorganisms from the microbiota of DFIs are frequently characterized as resistant to the standard antibiotics prescribed within general clinical practice (Mendes, et al. 2012). Both *S. aureus* and *P. aeruginosa* are well-known for their increased resistance to most conventional antibiotic agents, and the infections caused by antibiotic-resistant strains represent a serious threat to public health (Hancock and Speert 2000, Lowy 2003, Chambers and DeLeo 2009, Chatterjee, et al. 2016). Diabetic patients are a particular high-risk group, since the morbidity and mortality of patients with DFIs caused by resistant strains are significantly higher than those caused by non-resistant strains (Tascini 2018).

Both *S. aureus* and *P. aeruginosa* are also known for their ability to produce several virulence factors, namely protein and carbohydrate adhesins, exotoxins, exoenzymes and proteins involved in immune system evasion. The interaction of pathogens within the DFI polymicrobial biofilms favors the expression of quorum-sensing molecules, hemolysins, collagenases, proteases and short-chain fatty acids, responsible for inflammation and wound healing impeding, ultimately leading to DFI chronicity (Citron, et al. 2007, Hauser 2011, Oogai, et al. 2011, Jenkins, et al. 2015).

Staphylococci, particularly *S. aureus*, are perhaps the most virulent pathogens in DFIs, presenting a correlation between specific virulence genotypic markers and ulcer outcome (Sotto, et al. 2008). The overall burden of staphylococcal disease, particularly the one caused by methicillin-resistant *S. aureus* (MRSA) strains, is increasing in many countries (Mottola, Semedo-Lemsaddek, et al. 2016, Akhi, et al. 2017). Portugal presents one of the highest prevalence of diabetes *mellitus*-associated lower limb amputations (Carinci, et al. 2016) and MRSA skin and soft tissue infections in Europe (Moet, et al. 2007). Among hospitalized diabetic patients, the prevalence of MRSA in DFIs can range from 15 to 30% (Hobizal and Wukich 2012). *S. aureus* infections, particularly those affecting diabetic patients, are associated with severe consequences, since they can evolve from minor skin and soft tissue infections to extremely serious systemic diseases, such as endocarditis, septicemia and osteomyelitis (Jenkins, et al. 2015).

BIOFILM MODE OF GROWTH

DFIs are predominantly polymicrobial and their microorganisms can exhibit different modes of growth. DFI bacterial cells can be present in a non-adherent planktonic form, or they can form sessile microbial communities, irreversibly attached to surfaces, encaged within a self-produced matrix of extracellular polymeric substances, called biofilms (Dickschat 2010, Banu, et al. 2015).

In the DFI environment, the majority of bacterial cells are naturally organized in biofilms (Banu, et al. 2015, Mottola, Mendes, et al. 2016). This biofilm-forming ability is an important virulence factor presented by these pathogens and has been associated with resilient chronic foot wound infections that respond unsuccessfully to antibiotic therapy (James, et al. 2008, Banu, et al. 2015). Bacteria within biofilms are sheltered from numerous stressful conditions and the increased resistance to conventional antibiotics along with the recurrence presented by DFIs is a direct consequence of the multiple resistance mechanisms that biofilm-related bacteria possess (Batoni, Maisetta and Esin 2016).

The deleterious effect of the biofilm mode of microbial growth on wound healing has been known for decades (James, et al. 2008). These slime-enclosed aggregates of bacteria are characterized for being a very hostile environment for an efficient immune system response, as well as for antimicrobial agents penetration and diffusion (Hall and Mah 2017). Moreover, biofilm-based bacterial cells are physiologically distinct from non-adherent planktonic cells. Their growth rate is reduced and the quorum-sensing signaling system enables biofilm cells to activate specific genetic determinants of antibiotic tolerance and resistance (Dickschat 2010, Hall and Mah 2017), which can increase antibiotic resistance by up to 1000 fold (Stewart and Costerton 2001). Acting in concert, these mechanisms are responsible for the emergence of antibiotic-resistant strains and for biofilm recalcitrance, which is a major issue in the re-occurrence and delayed healing of infected chronic wounds, such as those presented by diabetic patients (Burmølle, et al. 2006, Lipsky, Aragón-Sánchez, et al. 2016).

INHIBITORY POTENTIAL OF ANTIMICROBIAL PEPTIDES

Over the last decades, antimicrobial peptides (AMPs) have attracted considerable interest as a new class of antimicrobial agents (Strempel, Strehmel and Overhage 2015, Pletzer, Coleman and Hancock 2016, Mahlapuu, et al. 2016). Considering the dissemination of bacterial resistance and the failure of conventional antibiotic-based therapies amongst diabetic patients, it is crucial to develop alternative treatment strategies, and AMPs are emerging as potential new weapons against these chronically infected wounds (Strempel, Strehmel and Overhage 2015, Pletzer, Coleman and Hancock 2016, Mahlapuu, et al. 2016).

Since DFI are caused by a diverse community of biofilm-producing bacteria, when managing these persistent infected wounds it is essential to use antimicrobial agents whose spectrum of activity covers both planktonic bacteria and sessile polymicrobial communities present in the DFI environments (Lipsky, Aragón-Sánchez, et al. 2016). For that reason, the development of new therapeutic strategies, namely the ones based on AMPs administration, which by their own or in a combination with other antimicrobial agents may target different elements of the DFI microbiota, might prove to be successful in the treatment and management of these infections.

AMPs are part of the innate immune defense system of virtually all living organisms, including bacteria, protozoan, fungi, plants, insects and animals (Bahar and Ren 2013, Mahlapuu, et al. 2016). These peptides are characterized by a low molecular weight, since they usually have less than one hundred amino acid residues; a cationic character, due to the high amount of positively charged residues; and an amphipathic structure, resulting from the presence of hydrophobic and hydrophilic regions in opposite sides of these molecules (Shai 1999, Wu, et al. 1999, Aoki and Ueda 2013).

Considering their polypeptide backbone, AMPs are commonly classified based on their structural characteristics, including linear, α-helical and β-hairpin-like structures (Zasloff 2002). Linear AMPs include indolicin and PR-39 from mammals (Agerberth, et al. 1991, Selsted, et al. 1992) and type-A lantibiotics such as nisin from lactic acid bacteria (McAuliffe, Ross and Hill 2001); AMPs with an α-helical structure include magainins from frogs (Bevins and Zasloff 1990), cecropins from insects and mammals (Lee, et al. 1989) and cathelicidins from mammals (Bals, et al. 1998, Dürr, Sudheendra and Ramamoorthy 2006); and the β-hairpin-like AMPs include polyphemusin and tachyplesin from crabs (Powers, et al. 2006, Imura, et al. 2007) and α- and β-defensins from humans (Ganz, et al. 1985) (Dhople, Krukemeyer and Ramamoorthy 2006).

Since the isolation of the first AMP, gramicidin, from a soil *Bacillus* strain by Dubos in 1939, AMPs have received much attention as a potential class of antimicrobial agents (Dubos 1939), and to date, almost six thousand AMPs have already been discovered or synthesized (Zhao, et al. 2013). AMPs have been shown to function as the first line of defense against several pathogenic organisms, with demonstrated antimicrobial efficacy against Gram-positive and Gram-negative bacteria (Bahar and Ren 2013), anaerobic bacteria (Arzese, et al. 2003), fungi (Delattin, et al. 2017) and even viruses (Hsieh and Hartshorn 2016).

In addition to their direct antimicrobial activity, these small cationic peptides are multifunctional components of the innate immunity of their hosts also playing an important role in inflammation, immune activation and wound healing (Bahar and Ren 2013, Mahlapuu, et al. 2016).

AMPs can act as effector molecules of the immune defense mechanism, with several studies describing their ability to modulate the host's inflammatory response (Gaspar, Veiga and Castanho 2013). Some AMPs are able to impede the lipopolysaccharide-induced cytokine release by macrophages, reducing the inflammation that develops during an infection by Gram-negative bacteria (Zhang, Mann and Tsai 1999). Other AMPs are able to stimulate the inflammatory response by inducing the release of cytokines and growth factors; recruitment of neutrophils and macrophages and antigen presentation; and migration and proliferation of endothelial cells, fibroblasts and keratinocytes (Bowdish, Davidson and Hancock 2005, Lai and Gallo 2009). Moreover, some AMPs also play a role during the late phase of wound healing by acting on granulation tissue formation via stimulation of extracellular matrix biosynthesis, collagen production, neovascularization and angiogenesis (Mangoni, McDermott and Zasloff 2016). AMPs involvement in tissue remodeling have also been observed and occurs through modulation of the extracellular matrix and stimulation of myofibroblasts differentiation (Mangoni, McDermott and Zasloff 2016).

ANTIMICROBIAL PEPTIDES MECHANISMS OF ACTION

The mechanisms of action presented by AMPs are surprisingly diverse and different from those presented by conventional antibiotics (Friedrich, et al. 2000, Aoki and Ueda 2013). There are three major targets of AMPs in bacterial cells: the cell wall, including the outer membrane and the peptidoglycan layer; the plasma membrane; and the cytoplasmic components (Mahlapuu, et al. 2016). Despite their ability to penetrate the bacterial cells and repress intracellular processes, namely protein and nucleic-acids synthesis, protein folding and enzymatic activity (Brogden 2005), it is well established that AMPs main mechanism of action is the disruption of microbial cell membranes (Mahlapuu, et al. 2016, Bechinger and Gorr 2017). Regardless of the differences in peptide sequence and structure, the majority of AMPs are highly cationic owing to the presence of a cluster of cationic amino acid residues (Shai 1999, Wu, et al. 1999, Aoki and Ueda 2013). Due to the highly content of negatively charged phospholipids, bacterial cell membranes are naturally attracted, through electrostatic forces, to cationic AMPs; on the contrary, eukaryotic cellular membranes, containing predominantly neutral phospholipids, tend to be unaffected by these small peptides. Moreover, the presence of cholesterol molecules in eukaryotic lipidic membranes also favors their resistance against AMPs disruption (Gottler and Ramamoorthy 2009).

Bacterial membrane disruption by AMPs can occur through diverse mechanisms, including pore formation in the lipid bilayer (barrel stave and toroidal pore models), membrane dissolution (carpet model), membrane thinning/thickening, lipid-peptide domain formation (micellization model), non-lytic membrane depolarization and electroporation (Nguyen, Haney and Vogel 2011, Gaspar, Veiga and Castanho 2013).

As previously mentioned, the formation of surface-attached and matrix-protected microbial biofilms and the slow growth rate and reduced metabolic activity presented by biofilm-encased bacterial cells are directly related to bacterial resistance towards antibiotics and innate immune system molecules (Burmølle, et al. 2006, James, et al. 2008). On the other hand, AMPs mainly exert their antibacterial activity by disrupting and permeating cell membranes, i. e, they present a mechanism of action that is independent of the bacterial metabolic state (Nguyen, Haney and Vogel 2011, Mahlapuu, et al. 2016, Bechinger and Gorr 2017). Considering that membrane integrity is essential for bacterial survival, this feature allows AMPs to be effective against metabolic active and dormant microbial cells, both co-existing in the polymicrobial environment of mature biofilms

(Strempel, Strehmel and Overhage 2015, Pletzer, Coleman and Hancock 2016).

Due to their mechanism of action AMPs generally induce a fast-killing-kinetics of bacterial cells. They are able to interact with the microbial cells and exert their activity in a short time frame, inducing a rapid bacterial death and decreasing the probability of resistance development (Fernebro 2011).

ANTIMICROBIAL PEPTIDES RESISTANCE

AMPs play a key role on host immunity by being one of its most old and efficient defense mechanisms. Possibly due to their different modes of action, bacteria have still not developed highly effective resistance mechanisms, such as those that impair the action of many therapeutic antibiotics (Peschel and Sahl 2006). In fact, while conventional antibiotics usually present a single defined primary target and a single mode of action, acting on specific components of the microbial cells to which they have a high affinity, AMPs molecules exert multiple antimicrobial activities, aiming at less specific cellular targets and affecting numerous biological functions (Yeaman and Yount 2003, Wang, et al. 2016).

While rarely observed, there are reports of resistance towards AMPs by bacterial pathogens. Resistance occurs through several mechanisms, namely proteolytic cleavage of AMPs due to the release of extracellular proteases, AMP-specific binding and extrusion via efflux pumps and alteration of the bacterial surface, specifically regarding surface molecules charges which contribute to decrease their affinity with AMPs. Nevertheless, AMPs resistance is limited and significantly reduced when compared to conventional antibiotics (Yeaman and Yount 2003, Park, Park and Hahm 2011).

The multiple modes of action presented by these peptides and the targeting of vital bacterial structures, such as the cytoplasmic membrane, are amongst the main reasons impairing the bacterial development of stable and competent AMPs resistance mechanisms (Yeaman and Yount 2003,

Fernebro 2011, Park, Park and Hahm 2011, Jorge, et al. 2017). Also, as the mechanisms responsible for AMPs resistance are diverse and different from antibiotic resistance mechanisms (Park, Park and Hahm 2011), cross-resistance between antibiotics and AMPs is rare, as demonstrated in a recent study by Lázár and colleagues that showed that antibiotic-resistant *Escherichia coli* strains present high susceptibility towards AMPs. These results support the hypothesis of the use of AMPs in combination with currently used antibiotics in order to control the emergence of multidrug-resistant bacteria (Lázár, et al. 2018).

ANTIMICROBIAL PEPTIDES IN THE DIABETIC FOOT INFECTION MANAGEMENT

The biomedical properties of AMPs support their potential as a new therapeutic approach to manage antibiotic-resistant infections, including DFIs. An acceptable antimicrobial agent to be used in DFI management should present activity against the broad-spectrum of bacteria in the DFI environment, limited toxicity in order to avoid serious adverse effects and low risk of resistance development. The growing interest in AMPs is not only due to the above-mentioned characteristics, but also to their immunomodulatory properties (Batoni, Maisetta and Esin 2016, Mahlapuu, et al. 2016). Also, many studies have demonstrated the antimicrobial activity of these molecules against both Gram-positive and Gram-negative bacteria and their ability to interfere with different stages of the biofilm growth mode (Park, Park and Hahm 2011, Batoni, Maisetta and Esin 2016, Pletzer, Coleman and Hancock 2016). Among the AMPs with potential to be applied in DFI treatment, nisin and pexiganan are two of the most promising ones.

Nisin is a class I bacteriocin, produced by *Lactococcus lactis*, and one of the most widely studied AMPs (Abts, et al. 2011, Zhu, Liua and Niu 2017). In 1969, this small polypeptide was considered safe for use as a food preservative by the Food and Agriculture Organization and World

Health Organization. Later, in 1983, nisin was added to the European list of food additives under the code E234 and five years later it was also approved by the United States Food and Drug Administration as "Generally Regarded As Safe" for use in pasteurized products and processed cheeses to inhibit the growth of *Clostridium botulinum* and *Listeria monocytogenes* (Jozala, Novaes and Junior 2015). The safety and efficacy of nisin as a food preservative have resulted in its widespread use throughout the world. Nowadays, nisin is used in over 48 countries (Jozala, Novaes and Junior 2015).

Nisin is a ribosomally synthesized, linear polypeptide containing 34 amino acid residues and with a molecular weight of 3500 Da. For presenting the unusual amino acid lanthionine in its structure, nisin is classified as a lantibiotic (Hansen 1994, McAuliffe, Ross and Hill 2001). Besides lanthionine and methyl-lanthionine, dehydroalanine and dehydrobutyrine, amino acids that are rarely found in nature, are also present on nisin's sequence and can be responsible for its antimicrobial activity and biophysical properties such as thermostability and solubility (McAuliffe, Ross and Hill 2001). The cationic nature of nisin is mainly due to the presence of lysine and histidine amino acid residues, while its amphipathicity is due to the presence of hydrophobic and hydrophilic amino acid residues at the N-terminal and C-terminal regions, respectively (McAuliffe, Ross and Hill 2001). Nisin biophysical properties are pH-dependent, presenting an increased solubility and stability under acidic conditions. In neutral or alkaline environments nisin tends to lose its efficiency (McAuliffe, Ross and Hill 2001).

Nisin has been shown to present a strong antimicrobial activity against a broad spectrum of Gram-positive bacteria and stable resistance is rarely reported (Zhu, Liua and Niu 2017). In fact, the long-term use of nisin in food industry does not seem to have prompted significant bacterial resistance towards this AMP (Bechinger and Gorr 2017). Nisin's spectrum of activity includes a wide range of Gram-positive bacteria, such as Staphylococci, Streptococci, Enterococci, Bacilli and Micrococci (Arauz, et al. 2009, Jozala, Novaes and Junior 2015, Zhu, Liua and Niu 2017). This peptide exerts its antimicrobial activity through a dual mode of action:

inhibition of cell wall synthesis and pore formation in the bacterial cytoplasmic membrane. Both mechanisms result from its interaction with the membrane-anchored peptidoglycan precursor lipid II, which is simultaneously used as a target and a pore constituent. Pore formation by nisin binding to lipid II molecules leads to efflux of cellular constituents, ultimately resulting in microbial death (Wiedemann, et al. 2001).

Nisin has also demonstrated ability to inhibit and kill biofilm-associated *S. aureus*, including some antibiotic resistant strains, isolated from infected diabetic foot ulcers (Santos, et al. 2016). However, the use of nisin as mono-therapeutic option to treat DFI can be limited. Indeed, the activity of nisin against Gram-negative organisms is much lower than its activity against peptidoglycan-rich Gram-positive bacteria (Breukink and Kruijff 1999, Li, Montalban-Lopez and Kuipersa 2018). A possible reason for this constraint is the fact that lipid II is predominantly located at the inner membrane of Gram-negative cells and their considerably impermeable outer membrane impedes nisin from reaching these molecules (Li, Montalban-Lopez and Kuipersa 2018). In order to overcome this limitation, nisin could be combined with a different AMP whose spectrum of action includes Gram-negative bacteria, such as pexiganan.

Pexiganan is a synthetic 22 amino acids residues peptide, analogue of magainin, co-discovered in 1987 by Zasloff (Zasloff 1987) and Giovannini and colleagues (Giovannini, et al. 1987). These scientists found out that this cationic small peptide, present in the skin secretion of the South African clawed frog *Xenopus laevis*, was directly related to its ability to resist microbial infections (Giovannini, et al. 1987, Zasloff 1987). Magainin is a water soluble polypeptide, containing 23 amino acid residues and a molecular mass of 2500 Da (Giovannini, et al. 1987) and has a broad-spectrum antimicrobial activity against various species of bacteria, fungi and protozoa (Zasloff, Martin and Chen 1988). Despite its well-known antimicrobial properties, magainin high non-specific toxicity makes its therapeutic application difficult. For that reason, its structure and activity have been widely studied and modifications have been introduced in order to reduce its toxicity towards animal cells and improve the antimicrobial activity of the related synthetic AMP, pexiganan (Zhu, Liua and Niu 2017). More specifically, single amino acid modifications were introduced with the aim of increasing the electrostatic attraction between this AMP and the negatively charged bacterial membranes (Gottler and Ramamoorthy 2009). Substitutions between the amino acid residues glycine and alanine increased the stability of the pexiganan α-helical structure, leading to an increased antimicrobial activity (Chen, et al. 1988).

It is believed that pexiganan exerts its antibacterial effect by disturbing the permeability of the bacterial cell membranes via toroidal pore formation. Specifically, pexiganan binds to the negatively charged bacterial lipid bilayers and forms an antiparallel dimer of amphipathic α-helices (Gottler and Ramamoorthy 2009). The toroidal pore mechanism is characterized by the bending of the cellular membrane, resulting in the formation of pores whose surface is formed by the lipid head groups (Gottler and Ramamoorthy 2009).

Pexiganan presents activity against a wide range of bacterial species. In a study conducted by Ge and colleagues, this AMP demonstrated an excellent *in vitro* activity against numerous bacterial species, including Gram-positive and Gram-negative aerobes and anaerobes isolated from diabetic patients with infected DFUs (Ge, Macdonald and Henry, et al. 1999). Pexiganan's activity against DFI isolates, namely *Staphylococcus* spp. including *S. aureus*, *Streptococcus* spp., *Enterococcus* spp., *Pseudomonas* spp. including *P. aeruginosa*, *Stenotrophomonas* spp., *Acinetobacter* spp., *Citrobacter* spp., *Bacteroides* spp., *Peptoniphilus* spp. and *Clostridium* spp. prompted its potential as a novel antimicrobial agent with promising therapeutic applications (Ge, Macdonald and Henry, et al. 1999, Ge, Macdonald and Holroyd, et al. 1999). Additionally, Ge al collegues also reported that the repeated contact with subinhibitory pexiganan concentrations did not generate resistant mutants and that cross-resistance with commonly used antibiotics, such as beta-lactams, quinolones, macrolides and lincosamides, was not observed (Ge, Macdonald and Holroyd, et al. 1999).

Pexiganan was the first AMP to be considered for commercial development aiming DFI treatment, and several clinical trials involving patients with infected DFU were conducted to evaluate its therapeutic potential (Gordon and Romanowski 2005, Mangoni, McDermott and Zasloff 2016). Regardless of excellent *in vitro* results, clinical trials results were not satisfactory. Pexiganan did not meet the primary clinical endpoint, since it did not produce any significant improvement in wound closure when compared to the topical placebo. Neither met the secondary endpoint of demonstrating a higher rate of bacterial eradication. Following these results, FDA approval was denied (Dipexium Pharmaceuticals 2017).

CONCLUSION

The prevalence of diabetes *mellitus* and DFIs related complications have drastically increased globally (World Health Organization 2016). Due to the high incidence of multidrug-resistant microorganisms in DFIs and the ineffectiveness of conventional antibiotic-based therapies, diabetic patients are at increased risk of developing the severe consequences of recalcitrant DFIs, namely wound inflammation, infection chronicity, foot gangrene, ultimately leading to lower-limb amputation (Hobizal and Wukich 2012, Lipsky, Aragón-Sánchez, et al. 2016). The emergence and dissemination of multidrug-resistant pathogens is a major global medical challenge, and diabetic patients therapeutics is no exception (Lipsky, Aragón-Sánchez, et al. 2016). Indeed, the biofilm forming ability and the antibiotic-resistance profile presented by numerous DFI isolates are accountable for the frightening scenario faced by these patients (Mendes, et al. 2012, Mottola, Mendes, et al. 2016).

Over the last decades, AMPs have emerged as a potential new answer to solve this problematic situation (Strempel, Strehmel and Overhage 2015, Pletzer, Coleman and Hancock 2016) and there are high expectations regarding the future of these peptides as alternative antimicrobial agents. In addition to their demonstrated antimicrobial activity against a wide range of pathogenic bacteria, these molecules are also able to modulate the host inflammatory response (Bahar and Ren 2013, Mahlapuu, et al. 2016).

Nisin and pexiganan are two of the most promising AMPs for application in the management of DFIs. These AMPs are amongst the most studied ones and are under research as potential therapeutics against DFI pathogens, including *S. aureus* and *P. aeruginosa* (Brumfitt, Salton and Hamilton-Miller 2002, Field, O' Connor, et al. 2016, Field, Seisling, et al. 2016, Flamm, et al. 2016, Santos, et al. 2016, van Staden, et al. 2016). However, previous studies suggest that these peptides present some limitations that need to be overcome. The development of combined therapeutics involving different antimicrobial agents may be one possible solution to surpass the limitations of pexiganan to act on DFIs *in vivo* (Dipexium Pharmaceuticals 2017) and the reduced activity of nisin against Gram-negative bacteria (Breukink and Kruijff 1999, Li, Montalban-Lopez and Kuipersa 2018).

AMPs can be used as antimicrobial agents alone or in combination with conventional antibiotics or other AMPs with different mechanisms and activity spectrum, in order to promote additive or synergistic effects (Pletzer, Coleman and Hancock 2016). Indeed, it is well established that synergistic interactions between antimicrobial molecules could decrease antimicrobial resistance and toxicity, improving their therapeutic potential (Pletzer, Coleman and Hancock 2016). The consensus among the scientific community is that AMPs exert their activity mostly through disruption of bacterial membranes (Gaspar, Veiga and Castanho 2013, Mahlapuu, et al. 2016, Bechinger and Gorr 2017). Microbial loss of membrane integrity promotes the entrance into the cell of antimicrobial agents, which makes AMPs efficient molecules to be used together with conventional antibiotics that have intracellular targets (Grassi, et al. 2017). In the literature there are numerous reports regarding the synergistic and additive effect of combinations between AMPs, such as nisin and pexiganan, and other antibacterial agents, reflecting their predisposition to be used as adjuvants of conventional antibiotic therapies (Garbacz, Kamysz and Piechowicz 2017, Jorge, et al. 2017).

The promising results obtained in the studies developed so far (Field, O' Connor, et al. 2016, Field, Seisling, et al. 2016) point out for the importance of further investigations regarding the use of AMPs against microbial pathogens, such as those present in DFIs. In conclusion, this chapter reinforces the need for a paradigm shift in antimicrobial treatment strategies by highlighting the potential use of AMPs as novel therapeutic weapons against antibiotic-resistant and biofilm-forming pathogens.

ACKNOWLEDGMENTS

Authors would like to acknowledge FCT – Fundação para a Ciência e a Tecnologia for the support of Project PTDC/SAU-INF/28466/2017 and Raquel Santos PhD fellowship SFRH/BD/100571/2014. Authors would also like to acknowledge Professor Ana Salomé Veiga for the critical review of the manuscript.

REFERENCES

Abts, André., Antonino, Mavaro., Jan, Stindt., Patrick, J. Bakkes., Sabine, Metzger., Arnold, J. Driessen., Sander, H. Smits. & Lutz, Schmitt. (2011). "Easy and Rapid Purification of Highly Active Nisin." *International Journal of Peptides*, *2011* (1), 1-9. doi:10.1155/2011/175145.

Agerberth, Birgitta., Joung-Youn, Lee., Tomas, Bergman., Mats, Carlquist., Hans, G. Boman., Viktor, Mutt. & Hans, Jörnvall. (1991). "Amino Acid Sequence of PR-39. Isolation from Pig Intestine of a New Member of the Family of Proline-Arginine-Rich Antibacterial Peptides." *European Journal of Biochemistry*, *202* (3), 849-854. doi:10.1111/j.1432-1033.1991.tb16442.x

Akhi, Mohammad., Reza, Ghotaslou., Mohammad, Memar., Mohammad, Asgharzadeh., Mojtaba, Varshochi., Tahereh, Pirzadeh. & Naser, Alizadeh. (2017). "Frequency of MRSA in Diabetic Foot Infections." *International Journal of Diabetes in Developing Countries*, *37* (1), 58-62. doi:10.1007/s13410-016-0492-7.

Aoki, Wataru. & Mitsuyoshi, Ueda. (2013). "Characterization of Antimicrobial Peptides Toward the Development of Novel Antibiotics." *Pharmaceuticals*, *6* (8), 1055-1081. doi:10.3390/ph6081055.

Arauz, Luciana., Angela, Jozala., Priscila, Mazzola. & Thereza, Penna. (2009). "Nisin Biotechnological Production and Application: A Review." *Trends in Food Science & Technology*, *20* (3), 146-154. doi:10.1016/j.tifs.2009.01.056.

Armstrong, David G., Kelman, Cohen., Stephane, Courric., Manish, Bharara. & William, Marston. (2011). "Diabetic Foot Ulcers and Vascular Insufficiency: Our Population Has Changed, but Our Methods Have Not." *Journal of Diabetes Science and Technology*, *5* (6), 1591-1595. doi:10.1177/193229681100500636.

Arzese, Alessandra., Barbara, Skerlavaj., Linda, Tomasinsig., Renato, Gennaro. & Margherita, Zanetti. (2003). "Antimicrobial Activity of SMAP-29 Against the *Bacteroides fragilis* Group and Clostridia." *Journal of Antimicrobial Chemotherapy*, *52* (3), 375-381. doi:10.1093/jac/dkg372.

Bahar, Ali Adem. & Dacheng, Ren. (2013). "Antimicrobial Peptides." *Pharmaceuticals*, *6* (12), 1543-1575. doi:10.3390/ph6121543.

Bals, Robert., Xiaorong, Wang., Michael, Zasloff. & James, Wilson. (1998). "The Peptide Antibiotic LL-37/hCAP-18 is Expressed in Epithelia of the Human Lung Where It Has Broad Antimicrobial Activity at the Airway Surface." *Proceedings of the National Academy of Sciences of the United States of America*, *95* (16), 9541-9546.

Banu, Asima., Mir, Mohammad., Noorul, Hassan., Janani, Rajkumar. & Sathyabheemarao, Srinivasa. (2015). "Spectrum of Bacteria Associated with Diabetic Foot Ulcer and Biofilm Formation: A Prospective Study." *Australasian Medical Journal*, *8* (9), 280-285. doi:10.4066/AMJ.2015.2422.

Batoni, Giovanna., Giuseppantonio, Maisetta. & Semih, Esin. (2016). "Antimicrobial Peptides and Their Interaction with Biofilms of Medically Relevant Bacteria." *Biochimica et Biophysica Acta*, *1858*, (5), 1044-1060. doi:10.1016/j.bbamem.2015.10.013.

Bechinger, Burkhard. & Sven-Ulrik, Gorr. (2017). "Antimicrobial Peptides: Mechanisms of Action and Resistance." *Journal of Dental Research*, 96 (3), 254-260. doi:10.1177/0022034516679973.

Bevins, Charles L. & Michael, Zasloff. (1990). "Peptides From Frog Skin." *Annual Review of Biochemistry*, 59, 395-414. doi:10.1146/annurev.bi.59.070190.002143.

Bowdish, Dawn., Donald, Davidson. & Robert, Hancock. (2005). "A Re-Evaluation of the Role of Host Defence Peptides in Mammalian Immunity." *Current Protein & Peptide Science*, 6 (1), 35-51.

Breukink, Eefjan. & Ben, de Kruijff. (1999). "The Lantibiotic Nisin, a Special Case or Not?" *Biochimica et Biophysica Acta*, 1462, 223-234.

Brogden, Kim A. (2005). "Antimicrobial Peptides: Pore Formers or Metabolic Inhibitors in Bacteria?" *Nature Reviews Microbiology*, 3 (3), 238-250. doi:10.1038/nrmicro1098.

Brumfitt, William., Milton, Salton. & Jeremy, Hamilton-Miller. (2002). "Nisin, Alone and Combined With Peptidoglycan-Modulating Antibiotics: Activity Against Methicillin-Resistant *Staphylococcus aureus* and Vancomycin-Resistant Enterococci." *Journal of Antimicrobial Chemotherapy*, 50 (5), 731-734. doi:10.1093/jac/dkf190.

Burmølle, Mette., Jeremy, S. Webb., Dhana, Rao., Lars, H. Hansen., Søren, J. Sørensen. & Staffan, Kjelleberg. (2006). "Enhanced Biofilm Formation and Increased Resistance to Antimicrobial Agents and Bacterial Invasion Are Caused by Synergistic Interactions in Multispecies Biofilms." *Applied and Environmental Microbiology*, 72 (6), 3916-3923. doi:10.1128/AEM.03022-05.

Carinci, Fabrizio., Massimo, M. Benedetti., Nicolaas, S. Klazinga. & Luigi, Uccioli. (2016). "Lower Extremity Amputation Rates in People with Diabetes as an Indicator of Health Systems Performance. A Critical Appraisal of the Data Collection 2000–2011 by the Organization for Economic Cooperation and Development (OECD)." *Acta Diabetologica*, 53 (5), 825-832. doi:10.1007/s00592-016-0879-4.

Chambers, Henry F. & Frank, R. DeLeo. (2009). "Waves of Resistance, *Staphylococcus aureus* in the Antibiotic Era." *Nature Reviews Microbiology*, 7 (9), 629-641. doi:10.1038/nrmicro2200.

Chatterjee, Maitrayee., Anju, Pushkaran., Lalitha, Biswas., Anil, Vasudevan., Chethampadi, Mohan. & Raja, Biswas. (2016). "Antibiotic Resistance in *Pseudomonas aeruginosa* and Alternative Therapeutic Options." *International Journal of Medical Microbiology*, 306 (1), 48-58. doi:10. 1016/j.ijmm.2015.11.004.

Chen, Hao-Chia., Judith, H. Brown., John, L. Morell. & Charng-Ming, Huang. (1988). "Synthetic Magainin Analogues With Improved Antimicrobial Activity." *FEBS Letters*, 236 (2), 462-466.

Citron, Diane M., Ellie, J. C. Goldstein., Vreni, Merriam., Benjamin, A. Lipsky. & Murray, A. Abramson. (2007). "Bacteriology of Moderate-to-Severe Diabetic Foot Infections and *in vitro* Activity of Antimicrobial Agents." *Journal of Clinical Microbiology*, 45 (9), 2819-2828. doi:10.1128/JCM.00551-07.

Delattin, Nicolas., Katrijn, Brucker., Kaat, Cremer., Bruno, Cammue. & Karin, Thevissen. (2017). "Antimicrobial Peptides as a Strategy to Combat Fungal Biofilms." *Current Topics in Medicinal Chemistry*, 17 (5), 604-612. doi: 10.2174/1568026616666160713142228.

Dhople, Vishnu., Amy, Krukemeyer. & Ayyalusamy, Ramamoorthy. (2006). "The Human Beta-defensin-3, an Antibacterial Peptide with Multiple Biological Functions." *Biochimica et Biophysica Acta*, 1758 (9), 1499-1512. doi:10.1016/j.bbamem.2006.07.007.

Dickschat, Jeroen S. (2010). "Quorum Sensing and Bacterial Biofilms." *Natural Product Reports*, 27 (3), 343-369. doi:10.1039/b804469b.

Dipexium, Pharmaceuticals. (2017). "Pexiganan Versus Placebo Control for the Treatment of Mild Infections of Diabetic Foot Ulcers." *Clinical Trials U. S. National Library of Medicine.*, 14, 06. Accès le 02 05, 2019. https://clinicaltrials.gov/ct2/show/NCT01590758.

Dubos, René J. (1939). "Studies on a Bactericidal Agent Extracted From a Soil *Bacillus*: I. Preparation of the Agent. Its Activity *in vitro*." *Journal of Experimental Medicine*, 70 (1), 1-10.

Dürr, Ulrich., Umar, Sudheendra. & Ayyalusamy, Ramamoorthy. (2006). "LL-37, the Only Human Member of the Cathelicidin Family of Antimicrobial Peptides." *Biochimica et Biophysica Acta*, 1758 (9), 1408-1425. doi:10.1016/j.bbamem.2006.03.030.

Fernebro, Jenny. (2011). "Fighting Bacterial Infections - Future Treatment Options." *Drug Resistance Updates*, *14* (2), 125-139. doi:10.1016/j.drup.2011.02.001.

Field, Des., Nynke, Seisling., Paul, Cotter., Paul, Ross. & Colin, Hill. (2016). "Synergistic Nisin-Polymyxin Combinations for the Control of *Pseudomonas* Biofilm Formation." *Frontiers in Microbiology*, *7* (1713). doi:10.3389/fmicb.2016.01713.

Field, Des., Rory, O' Connor., Paul, Cotter., Paul, Ross. & Colin, Hill. (2016). "*In vitro* Activities of Nisin and Nisin Derivatives Alone and In Combination with Antibiotics against *Staphylococcus* Biofilms." *Frontiers in Microbiology*, *7* (508). doi:10.3389/fmicb.2016.00508.

Flamm, Robert K., Paul, R. Rhomberg., David, J. Farrell. & Ronald, N. Jones. (2016). "*In vitro* Spectrum of Pexiganan Activity; Bactericidal Action and Resistance Selection Tested Against Pathogens With Elevated MIC Values to Topical Agents." *Diagnostic Microbiology and Infectious Diseases*, *86*, 66-69. doi:10.1016/j.diagmicrobio.2016.06.012.

Friedrich, Carol L., Dianne, Moyles., Terry, J. Beveridge. & Robert, E. Hancock. (2000). "Antibacterial Action of Structurally Diverse Cationic Peptides on Gram-Positive Bacteria." *Antimicrobial Agents and Chemotherapy*, *44*, 2086-2092. doi:10.1128/AAC.44.8.2086-2092.2000.

Ganz, Tomas., Michael, Selsted., Dorothy, Szklarek., Sylvia, Harwig., Kathleen, Daher., Dorothy, Bainton. & Robert, Lehrer. (1985). "Defensins. Natural Peptide Antibiotics of Human Neutrophils." *Journal of Clinical Investigation*, *76* (4), 1427-1435. doi:10.1172/JCI112120.

Garbacz, Katarzyna., Wojciech, Kamysz. & Lidia, Piechowicz. (2017). "Activity of Antimicrobial Peptides, Alone or Combined With Conventional Antibiotics, Against *Staphylococcus aureus* Isolated From the Airways of Cystic Fibrosis Patients." *Virulence*, *8* (1), 94-100. doi:10.1080/21505594.2016.1213475.

Gaspar, Diana., Ana, Salomé Veiga. & Miguel, A. Castanho. (2013). "From Antimicrobial to Anticancer Peptides. A Review." *Frontiers in Microbiology*, *4* (294). doi:10.3389/fmicb.2013.00294.

Ge, Yigong., Dorothy, L. MacDonald., Kenneth, J. Holroyd., Clyde, Thornsberry., Hannah, Wexler. & Michael, Zasloff. (1999). "*In vitro* Antibacterial Properties of Pexiganan, an Analog of Magainin." *Antimicrobial Agents and Chemotherapy*, *43* (4), 782-788.

Ge, Yigong., Dorothy, L. MacDonald., Marietta, Henry., Howard, Hait., Kimberly, Nelson., Benjamin, A. Lipsky., Michael, A. Zasloff. & Kenneth, Holroyd. (1999). "*In vitro* Susceptibility to Pexiganan of Bacteria Isolated From Infected Diabetic Foot Ulcers." *Diagnostic Microbiology Infectius Disease*, *35* (1), 45-53. doi:10.1016/S0732-8893(99)00056-5.

Giovannini, Maria., Linda, Poulter., Bradford, Gibson. & Dudley, Williams. (1987). "Biosynthesis and Degradation of Peptides Derived From *Xenopus laevis* Prohormones." *The Biochemical Journal*, *243* (1), 113-120. doi:10.1042/bj2430113.

Gordon, Jerold. & Eric, Romanowski. (2005). "A Review of Antimicrobial Peptides and Their Therapeutic Potential as Anti-Infective Drugs." *Current Eye Research*, *30* (7), 505-515. doi:10.1080/02713680 590968637.

Gottler, Lindsey M. & Ayyalusamy, Ramamoorthy. (2009). "Structure, Membrane Orientation, Mechanism, and Function of Pexiganan – A Highly Potent Antimicrobial Peptide Designed From Magainin." *Biochimica et Biophysica Acta*, *1788* (8), 1680-1686. doi:10.1016/ j.bbamem.2008.10.009.

Grassi, Lucia., Giuseppantonio, Maisetta., Semih, Esin. & Giovanna, Batoni. (2017). "Combination Strategies to Enhance the Efficacy of Antimicrobial Peptides against Bacterial Biofilms." *Frontiers in Microbiology*, *8* (2409). doi:10.3389/fmicb.2017.02409.

Hall, Clayton W. & Thien-Fah, Mah. (2017). "Molecular Mechanisms of Biofilm-Based Antibiotic Resistance and Tolerance in Pathogenic Bacteria." *FEMS Microbiology Reviews*, *41* (3), 276-301. doi:10.1093/femsre/fux010.

Hancock, Robert E. W. & David, P. Speert. (2000). "Antibiotic Resistance in *Pseudomonas aeruginosa*: Mechanisms and Impact on Treatment." *Drug Resistance Updates*, *3* (4), 247-255. doi:10.1054/drup.2000.0152.

Hansen, John Norman. (1994). "Nisin as a Model Food Preservative." *Critical Reviews in Food Science and Nutrition*, *34* (1), 69-93. doi:10.1080/10408399409527650.

Hauser, Alan R. (2011). "*Pseudomonas aeruginosa*: So Many Virulence Factors, So Little Time." *Critical Care Medicine*, *39* (9), 2193-2194. doi:10.1097/CCM.0b013e318221742d.

Hobizal, Kimberlee B. & Dane, K. Wukich. (2012). "Diabetic Foot Infections: Current Concept Review." *Diabetic Foot & Ankle*, *3* (18409). doi:10.3402/dfa.v3i0.18409.

Hsieh, I-Ni. & Kevan, L. Hartshorn. (2016). "The Role of Antimicrobial Peptides in Influenza Virus Infection and Their Potential as Antiviral and Immunomodulatory Therapy." *Pharmaceuticals*, *9* (3). doi:10.3390/ph9030053.

Imura, Yuichi., Minoru, Nishida., Yoshiyuki, Ogawa., Yoshinobu, Takakura. & Katsumi, Matsuzaki. (2007). "Action Mechanism of Tachyplesin I and Effects of PEGylation." *Biochimica et Biophysica Acta*, *5*, 1160-1169. doi:10.1016/j.bbamem.2007.01.005.

James, Garth A., Ellen, Swogger., Randall, Wolcott., Elinor, deLancey Pulcini., Patrick, Secor., Jennifer, Sestrich., John, W. Costerton. & Philip, S. Stewart. (2008). "Biofilms in Chronic Wounds." *Wound Repair and Regeneration*, *16*, 37-44. doi:10.1111/j.1524-475X.2007.00321.

Jenkins, Amy., Binh, An Diep., Thuy, T. Mai., Nhung, H. Vo., Paul, Warrener., Joann, Suzich., Kendall, Stover. & Bret, R. Sellman. (2015). "Differential Expression and Roles of *Staphylococcus aureus* Virulence Determinants during Colonization and Disease." *mBio*, *6* (1). doi:10.1128/mBio.02272-14.

Jorge, Paula., Martín, Pérez-Pérez., Gael, Pérez Rodríguez., Maria, Olívia Pereira. & Anália, Lourenço. (2017). "A Network Perspective on Antimicrobial Peptide Combination Therapies: the Potential of

Colistin, Polymyxin B and Nisin." *International Journal of Antimicrobial Agents*, *49* (6), 668-676. doi:10.1016/j.ijantimicag.2017. 02.012.

Jozala, Angela., Letícia, Novaes. & Adalberto, Junior. (2015). "Nisin." In *Concepts, Compounds and the Alternatives of Antibacterials*, by Varaprasad Bobbarala, 103-120. IntechOpen. doi:10.5772/60932.

Kosinski, Mark A. & Benjamin, A Lipsky. (2010). "Current Medical Management of Diabetic Foot Infections." *Expert Review of Anti-infective Therapy*, *8* (11), 1293-1305. doi:10.1586/eri.10.122.

Lai, Yuping. & Richard, L. Gallo. (2009). "AMPed Up Immunity: How Antimicrobial Peptides Have Multiple Roles in Immune Defense." *Trends in Immunology*, *30* (3), 131-141. doi:10.1016/j.it.2008.12.003.

Lázár, Viktória., Ana, Martins., Réka, Spohn., Lejla, Daruka., Gábor, Grézal., Gergely, Fekete., Mónika, Számel., et al. (2018). "Antibiotic-Resistant Bacteria Show Widespread Collateral Sensitivity to Antimicrobial Peptides." *Nature Microbiology*, *3* (6), 718-731. doi:10.1038/s41564-018-0164-0.

Lee, J., Boman, A., Sun, C., Andersson, M., Jörnvall, H., Mutt, V. & Boman, H. (1989). "Antibacterial Peptides From Pig Intestine: Isolation of a Mammalian Cecropin." *Proceedings of the National Academy of Sciences of the United States of America*, *86* (23), 9159-9162. doi:10.1073/pnas.86.23.9159.

Li, Qian., Manuel, Montalban-Lopez. & Oscar, P. Kuipersa. (2018). "Increasing the Antimicrobial Activity of Nisin-Based Lantibiotics Against Gram-Negative Pathogens." *Applied and Environmental Microbiology*, *84* (12). doi:10.1128/AEM.00052-18.

Lipsky, Benjamin A., Anthony, R. Berendt., Paul, B. Cornia., James, C. Pile., Edgar, J. G. Peters., David, G. Armstrong., Gunner Deery, H., et al. (2012). "2012 Infectious Diseases Society of America Clinical Practice Guideline for the Diagnosis and Treatment of Diabetic Foot Infections." *Clinical Infectious Diseases*, *54* (12), 132-173. doi:10. 1093/cid/cis346.

Lipsky, Benjamin A., Javier, Aragón-Sánchez., Mathew, Diggle., John, Embil., Shigeo, Kono., Lawrence, Lavery., Éric, Senneville., et al.

(2016). "IWGDF Guidance on the Diagnosis and Management of Foot Infections in Persons with Diabetes." *Diabetes Metabolism Research and Reviews*, *32* (1), 45-74. doi:10.1002/dmrr.2699.

Lowy, Franklin D. (2003). "Antimicrobial Resistance: the Example of Staphylococcus aureus." *Journal of Clinical Investigation*, *111* (9), 1265-1273. doi:10.1172/JCI200318535.

Mahlapuu, Margit., Joakim, Håkansson., Lovisa, Ringstad. & Camilla, Björn. (2016). "Antimicrobial Peptides: An Emerging Category of Therapeutic Agents." *Frontiers in Cellular and Infection Microbiology*, *6* (197). doi:10.3389/fcimb.2016.00194.

Mangoni, Maria Luisa., Alison, M. McDermott. & Michael, Zasloff. (2016). "Antimicrobial Peptides and Wound Healing: Biological and Therapeutic Considerations." *Experimental Dermatology*, *25* (3), 167-173. doi:10.1111/exd.12929.

McAuliffe, Olivia., Paul Ross, R. & Colin, Hill. (2001). "Lantibiotics: Structure, Biosynthesis and Mode of Action." *FEMS Microbiology Reviews*, *25* (3), 285-308. doi:10.1111/j.1574-6976.2001.tb00579.x.

Mendes, João J., Ana, Marques-Costa., Cristina, Vilela., José, Neves., Nuno, Candeias., Patrícia, Cavaco-Silva. & José, Melo-Cristino. (2012). "Clinical and Bacteriological Survey of Diabetic Foot Infections in Lisbon." *Diabetes Research and Clinical Practice*, *95*, 153-161. doi:10.1016/j.diabres.2011.10.001.

Moet, Gary J., Ronald, N. Jones., Douglas, J. Biedenbacha., Matthew, G. Stilwell. & Thomas, R. Fritsche. (2007). "Contemporary Causes of Skin and Soft Tissue Infections in North America, Latin America, and Europe: Report from the SENTRY Antimicrobial Surveillance Program (1998-2004)." *Diagnostic Microbiology and Infectious Disease*, *57* (1), 7-13. doi:10.1016/j.diagmicrobio.2006.05.009.

Mottola, Carla., João, J. Mendes., José, Melo Cristino., Patrícia, Cavaco-Silva., Luís, Tavares. & Manuela, Oliveira. (2016). "Polymicrobial Biofilms By Diabetic Foot Clinical Isolates." *Folia Microbiologica*, *61* (1), 35-43. doi:10.1007/s12223-015-0401-3.

Mottola, Carla., Teresa, Semedo-Lemsaddek., João, J Mendes., José, Melo-Cristino., Luís, Tavares., Patrícia, Cavaco-Silva. & Manuela, Oliveira.

(2016). "Molecular Typing, Virulence Traits and Antimicrobial Resistance of Diabetic Foot Staphylococci." *Journal of Biomedical Science, 8*, 23-33. doi:10.1186/s12929-016-0250-7.

Nguyen, Leonard T., Evan, F. Haney. & Hans, J. Vogel. (2011). "The Expanding Scope of Antimicrobial Peptide Structures and Their Modes of Action." *Trends in Biotechnology, 29* (9), 464-472. doi:10.1016/j.tibtech.2011.05.001.

Oogai, Yuichi., Miki, Matsuo., Masahito, Hashimoto., Fuminori, Kato., Motoyuki, Sugai. & Hitoshi, Komatsuzawa. (2011). "Expression of Virulence Factors by *Staphylococcus aureus* Grown in Serum." *Applied and Environmental Microbiology, 77* (22), 8097-8105. doi:10.1128/AEM.05316-11.

Park, Seong-Cheol., Yoonkyung, Park. & Kyung-Soo, Hahm. (2011). "The Role of Antimicrobial Peptides in Preventing Multidrug-Resistant Bacterial Infections and Biofilm Formation." *International Journal of Molecular Sciences, 12* (9), 5971-5992. doi:10.3390/ijms12095971.

Peschel, Andreas. & Hans-Georg, Sahl. (2006). "The Co-evolution of Host Cationic Antimicrobial Peptides and Microbial Resistance." *Nature Reviews Microbiology, 4* (7), 529-536. doi:10.1038/nrmicro1441.

Pletzer, Daniel., Shannon, R. Coleman. & Robert, E. W. Hancock. (2016). "Anti-Biofilm Peptides as a New Weapon in Antimicrobial Warfare." *Current Opinion in Microbiology, 33*, 35-40. doi:10.1016/j.mib.2016.05.016.

Powers, Jon-Paul S., Morgan, M. Martin., Danika, L. Goosney. & Robert, E. W. Hancock. (2006). "The Antimicrobial Peptide Polyphemusin Localizes to the Cytoplasm of *Escherichia coli* Following Treatment." *Antimicrobial Agents and Chemotherapy, 50* (4), 1522-1524. doi:10.1128/AAC.50.4.1522-1524.2006.

Santos, Raquel., Diana, Gomes., Hermes, Macedo., Diogo, Barros., Catarina, Tibério., Ana, Salomé Veiga., Luís, Tavares., Miguel, Castanho. & Manuela, Oliveira. (2016). "Guar Gum as a New Antimicrobial Peptide Delivery System Against Diabetic Foot Ulcers *Staphylococcus aureus* Isolates." *Journal of Medical Microbiology, 65*, 1-8. doi:10.1099/jmm. 0.000329.

Selsted, Michael., Michael, Novotny., Wendy, Morris., Yi-Quan, Tang., Wayne, Smith. & James, Cullor. (1992). "Indolicidin, a Novel Bactericidal Tridecapeptide Amide from Neutrophils." *Journal of Biological Chemistry*, *267* (7), 4292-4295.

Shai, Yechiel. (1999). "Mechanism of the Binding, Insertion and Destabilization of Phospholipid Bilayer Membranes by Alpha-Helical Antimicrobial and Cell Non-Selective Membrane-Lytic Peptides." *Biochimica et Biophysica Acta*, *1462* (1), 55-70. doi:10.1016/S0005-2736(99)00200-X.

Sotto, Albert., Gérard, Lina., Jean-Louis, Richard., Christophe, Combescure., Gisèle, Bourg., Laure, Vidal., Nathalie, Jourdan., Jérôme, Etienne. & Jean-Philippe, Lavigne. (2008). "Virulence Potential of *Staphylococcus aureus* Strains Isolated From Diabetic Foot Ulcers." *Diabetes Care*, *31* (12), 2318-2324. doi:10.2337/dc08-1010.

Stewart, Philip S. & William Costerton, J. (2001). "Antibiotic Resistance of Bacteria in Biofilms." *Lancet*, *358*, 135-138. doi:10.1016/S0140-6736(01)05321-1

Strempel, Nikola., Janine, Strehmel. & Joerg, Overhage. (2015). "Potential Application of Antimicrobial Peptides in the Treatment of Bacterial Biofilm Infections." *Current Pharmaceutical Design*, *21* (1), 67-84. doi:10.2174/1381612820666140905124312

Tascini, Carlo. (2018). *Resistant Infections in the Diabetic Foot: A Frightening Scenario.*, Vol. 26, *The Diabetic Foot Syndrome*, by A Piaggesi and J Apelqvist, edited by M Porta, 161-166. Basel: Karger. doi:10.1159/000480061.

van Staden, Anton., Tiaan, Heunis., Carine, Smith., Shelly, Deane. & Leon, M. Dicks. (2016). "Efficacy of Lantibiotic Treatment of *Staphylococcus aureus*-Induced Skin Infections, Monitored by *in vivo* Bioluminescent Imaging." *Antimicrobial Agents Chemotherapy*, 60, 3948-3955. doi:10.1128/AAC.02938-15.

Wang, Shuai., Xiangfang, Zeng., Qing, Yang. & Shiyan, Qiao. (2016). "Antimicrobial Peptides as Potential Alternatives to Antibiotics in

Food Animal Industry." *International Journal of Molecular Sciences*, *17* (5). doi:10.3390/ijms17050603.

Wiedemann, Imke., Eefjan, Breukink., Cindy, van Kraaij., Oscar, P. Kuipers., Gabriele, Bierbaum., Ben, de Kruijff. & Hans-Georg, Sahl. (2001). "Specific Binding of Nisin to the Peptidoglycan Precursor Lipid II Combines Pore Formation and Inhibition of Cell Wall Biosynthesis for Potent Antibiotic Activity." *The Journal of Biological Chemistry*, *276* (1), 1772-1779. doi:10.1074/jbc.M006770200.

World Health Organization. (2016). *Global Report on Diabetes*. Geneva, Switzerland: Who Press.

Wu, Manhong., Elke, Maier., Roland, Benz. & Robert, E. W. Hancock. (1999). "Mechanism of Interaction of Different Classes of Cationic Antimicrobial Peptides with Planar Bilayers and with the Cytoplasmic Membrane of *Escherichia coli*." *Biochemistry*, *38* (22), 7235-7242. doi:10.1021/bi9826299.

Yazdanpanah, Leila., Morteza, Nasiri. & Sara, Adarvishi. (2015). "Literature Review on the Management of Diabetic Foot Ulcer." *World Journal of Diabetes*, *6* (1), 37-53. doi:10.4239/wjd.v6.i1.37.

Yeaman, Michael R. & Nannette, Y. Yount. (2003). "Mechanisms of Antimicrobial Peptide Action and Resistance." *The American Society for Pharmacology and Experimental Therapeutics*, *55* (1), 27-55. doi:10.1124/pr.55.1.2.

Zasloff, Michael. (1987). "Magainins, a Class of Antimicrobial Peptides From *Xenopus* Skin: Isolation, Characterization of Two Active Forms, and Partial cDNA Sequence of a Precursor." *Proceedings of the National Academy of Sciences of the United States of America*, *84* (15), 5449-5453. doi:10.1073/pnas.84.15.5449.

Zasloff, Michael. (2002). "Antimicrobial Peptides of Multicellular Organisms." *Nature*, *415* (6870), 389-395. doi:10.1038/415389a.

Zasloff, Michael., Brian, Martin. & Hao-Chia, Chen. (1988). "Antimicrobial Activity of Synthetic Magainin Peptides and Several Analogues." *Proceedings of the National Academy of Sciences of the United States of America*, *85* (3), 910-913. doi:10.1073/pnas.85.3.910.

Zhang, Gui-Hang., David, M. Mann. & Chao-Ming, Tsai. (1999). "Neutralization of Endotoxin *in vitro* and *in vivo* by a Human Lactoferrin-Derived Peptide." *Infection and Immunity*, *67* (3), 1353-1358.

Zhao, Xiaowei., Hongyu, Wu., Hairong, Lu., Guodong, Li. & Qingshan, Huang. (2013). "LAMP: A Database Linking Antimicrobial Peptides." *PLoS One*, *8* (6). doi:10.1371/journal.pone.0066557.

Zhu, Meng., Peng, Liua. & Zhong-Wei, Niu. (2017). "A Perspective on General Direction and Challenges Facing Antimicrobial Peptides." *Chinese Chemical Letters*, *28* (4), 703-708. doi:10.1016/j.cclet.2016.10.001.

In: Diabetic Foot: Prevention and Treatment ISBN: 978-1-53616-266-0
Editor: Gianni Romano © 2019 Nova Science Publishers, Inc.

Chapter 4

PROSPECTIVE ON ADVANCED DFU THERAPIES: IDENTIFYING ALTERNATIVES TO CONVENTIONAL THERAPY BASED ON CURRENT RESEARCH

Isa Serrano, Raquel Santos, Rui Soares, Luis Tavares and Manuela Oliveira[*]

CIISA - Centre for Interdisciplinary Research in Animal Health, Faculty of Veterinary Medicine University of Lisbon, Lisbon, Portugal

ABSTRACT

Diabetes *mellitus* (DM) is one of the most epidemic chronic diseases worldwide. From 1980 to 2014, there was a global increase of the disease prevalence, reaching 314 million adults aged over 18 years, a number which is expected to double by the year 2030. Recent studies show that diabetic patients have a 25% risk of developing diabetic foot ulcers (DFU) in their lifetime. Most (40-80%) DFU become infected, usually by polymicrobial populations, delaying wound healing and contributing to

---

[*] Corresponding Author's E-mail: moliveira@fmv.ulisboa.pt.

their chronicity. In 15% to 27% of the cases, DFU development leads to minor or major amputations of lower limbs, which in half of the cases are due to infection. As these amputations are a major cause of morbidity and mortality, new strategies to promote wound healing are urgent.

Several advanced DFU therapies are being developed and include novel antiseptics, bio-engineered skin, negative pressure wound therapy, electrical stimulation, recombinant human platelet-derived growth factor, hyperbaric oxygen therapy, granulocyte-colony stimulating factor, low-level light therapy, and bacteriophage therapy. From these, only bio-engineered skin and negative pressure are recommended for DFU treatment. This review will discuss advanced DFU therapies based on current research.

Keywords: diabetic foot ulcers, advanced therapies, antiseptics, bio-engineered skin, negative pressure wound therapy, electrical stimulation, recombinant human platelet-derived growth factor, hyperbaric oxygen therapy, granulocyte-colony stimulating factor, low-level light therapy, bacteriophage therapy

INTRODUCTION

Diabetes *mellitus* (DM) is one of the most epidemic chronic diseases worldwide. Several factors contribute to the increasing prevalence of DM, namely reduced physical activity, increased obesity, population growth, and aging. According to the World Health Organization (WHO), from 1980 to 2014 there was a global increase of the disease, from 4.7% to 8.5%, with 314 million adults aged over 18 years living with DM by that date. The majority of DM patients are affected by type 2 diabetes, more prevalent in adults, in comparison with type 1 diabetes, which is more threatful and not preventable. In type 2 diabetes the body cannot properly use the insulin it produces, whereas, in type 1 diabetes, patients do not produce enough insulin, requiring lifelong insulin injections for survival (WHO 2016). As a result of the increase in human longevity, diabetes prevalence is expected to double by 2030 if preventive measures are not adopted. In fact, this scenario may be even worst than predicted because of the increasing prevalence of obesity (Wild et al. 2004).

An overwhelming complication of diabetes is the development of diabetic foot ulcers (DFU). DFU are full-thickness wounds with skin necrosis or gangrene, below the ankle, induced by peripheral neuropathy or peripheral arterial disease in a diabetic patient, independently of its duration. Most DFU are chronic wounds that have not healed in 3 months (Chuan 2015).

A third of the patients with DFU are under 50 years of age, and its prevalence in the Western countries is of 4-10% (Gottrup 2005). In Canada and United States, diabetic patients have a 15-25% risk of developing DFU during their lifetime (Hobizal and Wukich 2012), and the annual incidence may be as high as 6% (Rice et al. 2014). After the first three months, only 10-60% of patients present healed ulcers. The recurrence rate of DFU is of 44% after one year, and of 61% and 70% after two and three years, respectively, resulting in repeated interventions and progressive disability (Gottrup 2005).

Between 15% to 27% of DFU cases require minor or major amputations of lower limbs, with infection being the preponderant factor in 50% of amputations (van Battum et al. 2011). Diabetic foot infections (DFI) are defined as infra-malleolar infections in a person with DM and are a common trait in DM patients, with a reported incidence between 40% and 80%. Diabetes-associated factors like hyperglycemia facilitate the development of infections and vice versa, creating a vicious cycle (Boyanova and Mitov 2013). The most common and classical lesion is *"mal perforans"* foot ulcer, which is characterized by a breach of the protective layer of skin, exposing the underlying tissues to bacterial colonization. Around 25% of the cases will spread from the epidermal layer to deeper regions, causing necrotic fasciitis, septic arthritis, and osteomyelitis (Noor, Zubair, and Ahmad 2015).

Generally, acute DFI in patients who have not recently been subjected to antibiotherapy are monomicrobial, whereas chronic infections are often polymicrobial (Noor, Zubair, and Ahmad 2015). Acute DFI are frequently caused by aerobic Gram-positive cocci, with *Staphylococcus aureus* being the most common pathogen (Noor, Zubair, and Ahmad 2015; Tascini

2011). Fungi have also been associated with diabetic foot wounds colonization and infection (Dowd et al. 2011).

As bacterial communities in DFI are often organized as polymicrobial biofilms, this trait limits the efficiency of antibiotic therapy and may be responsible for infection chronicity (Hobizal and Wukich 2012). Biofilm production is one of the most important virulence traits of *S. aureus*, particularly of methicillin-resistant *S. aureus* (MRSA), which as a prevalence of 15 to 30% in hospitalized patients with DFI (Eleftheriadou 2010; Hobizal and Wukich 2012). Diabetes is associated with immunological deficiencies, including abnormal neutrophil chemotaxis, phagocytosis, and intracellular death. These factors contribute to the reported clinical failure rates of 20% to 30% of foot infections treatment (Geerlings and Hoepelman 1999). In fact, nearly one in six patients die within 1 year after infection diagnose (Hobizal and Wukich 2012).

To assess the severity of a foot ulcer there are several standardized systems. SINBAD classifies ulcers according to a scoring system after assessing Site, Ischemia, Neuropathy, Bacterial Infection, Area and Depth of DFU (Ince et al. 2008). The University of Texas classification system assesses ulcer depth, presence of infection, signs of lower-extremity ischemia, allowing to classify ulcers in four grades and four stages (Armstrong, Lavery, and Harkless 1998). PEDIS classifies DFU according to five categories, depending on their Perfusion, Extent, Depth, Infection, and Sensation (Chuan et al. 2015). Finally, the Wagner classification classifies ulcers according to 5 grades: from grade 0 (no ulcer but high-risk foot) to grade 5 (extensive gangrene involving the whole foot) (NICE 2015). PEDIS predicts the clinical outcome more effectively, since the Wagner classification exclusively assesses ulcer depth, without considering co-morbidities such as ischemia and neuropathy (NICE 2015).

After assessing the severity of a foot ulcer, the conventional therapies in use include optimized control and management of blood glucose, foot care education, preventive foot care, limb elevation, ulcer debridement, offloading, antibiotic therapy, and surgical procedures (Mulder, Tenenhaus, and D'Souza 2014).

Optimized control and management of blood glucose levels aim to the early detection of abnormal blood glucose levels to proceed to adequate treatment. Although it may seem logical that the tight control of blood glucose levels would contribute to improve DFU healing, there are few data available regarding the relationship between the frequency of blood glucose measurements and DFU prognosis (Fernando et al. 2016).

Regarding foot care education, including preventive foot care and regular limb elevation, the few studies available revealed that a large proportion of the patients that need to be hospitalized for DFU treatment practice insufficient DFU self-management. Data suggest that diabetic foot self-care practice should be encouraged and patient education regarding foot care should be widespread (Chin et al. 2019).

Debridement is the removal of necrotic and senescent tissues as well as foreign and infected materials (Davis, Martinez, and Kirsner 2006). An efficient debridement should be carried along with adequate dressings, topical wound healing agents, or wound closure procedures (Yazdanpanah, Nasiri, and Adarvish 2015). Adequate dressings are chosen based on characteristics that include absorption, wound fluid removal, bacterial barrier, retention, and moisture maintenance (Mulder, Tenenhaus, and D'Souza 2014). Offloading is commonly known as pressure modulation. Predominantly, DFU will occur on the foot sole, being very important to off-load this area.

Offloading is considered a gold-standard component for the management of neuropathic ulcers and necessary for DFU healing (Armstrong et al. 2004; Yazdanpanah, Nasiri, and Adarvish 2015).

Antibiotic therapy is always relevant in the treatment of chronic DFI. However, systemic antibiotic therapy is associated with a high-risk of antibiotic resistance dissemination (Fair and Tor 2014). Bacterial high antimicrobial resistance profile combined with the presence of biofilm-producing strains limits the efficiency of antibiotic therapy. Furthermore, treatment efficiency is limited by the lack of blood supply to the wound surface. So, it is strongly recommended to perform a bacterial culture and antimicrobial susceptibility testing prior to starting empiric antibiotic therapy aiming at DFI treatment (Lipsky et al. 2012).

Surgical procedures for DFU healing include vascular and non-vascular foot surgery, but sometimes amputation is needed (Lipsky et al. 2004). To avoid limb amputation, it is important to: rapidly identify risk factors for DFI development; accurately classify these infections in order to guide treatment protocols; to have a multidisciplinary team involved in the evaluation of the foot infection; and reliable communication between health care providers (Hobizal and Wukich 2012).

Healing of a single ulcer costs approximately US$7500 (1998 currency), and extremity amputation is approximately US$14250 more expensive (Ragnarson and Apelqvist 2004). In addition, estimated losses in gross domestic product due to DM worldwide will total US$1.7 trillion between 2011 and 2030 (Bloom et al. 2011). Complementary advanced therapies may be used to promote wound healing and avoid amputation when conventional therapeutic protocols are not sufficient for the effective treatment of foot ulcers. The enormous investment in the development of new strategies responds to the challenging increase in DM and to the high social and economic burden associated with the disease (Yazdanpanah, Nasiri, and Adarvish 2015). The scaling-up of interventions that are cost-effective would significantly improve the quality of patients' lives and contribute to control the economic burden of DM (WHO 2016).

Several advanced therapies are commercially available, and many others are still in development. This review will focus on novel antiseptics, bio-engineered skin, negative pressure wound therapy, electrical stimulation, recombinant human platelet-derived growth factor, hyperbaric oxygen therapy, granulocyte-colony stimulating factor, low-level light therapy, and bacteriophage therapy.

In this review, advanced therapies for DFU chosen due to their relevance will be further discussed based on current research, highlighting their potential application, cost-effectiveness, as well as their advantages and drawbacks as complementary treatments to conventional therapies. Nowadays, regulatory and policy constraints limit the use of bacteriophage therapy for DFI treatment, and this issue will also be further addressed.

ADVANCED THERAPEUTICS

The National Institute for Health and Care Excellence (NICE), England, has elaborated recommendations to each advanced therapy which are summarized in Table 1.

Table 1. Recommendations of the National Institute for Health and Care Excellence (NICE) on advanced therapies for the treatment of diabetic foot ulcers

Advanced therapies	NICE recommendation
Dermal or skin substitutes	Should be used as a complement to standard care only when healing has not progressed and with the guidance of a multidisciplinary foot care service.
Negative pressure	Should be applied after surgical debridement, on the advice of the multidisciplinary foot care service.
Electrical stimulation; Recombinant human platelet-derived growth factor; Hyperbaric oxygen therapy; Granulocyte-colony stimulating factor	Should not be used as complementary treatment for in-hospital patients, unless as part of a clinical trial.

Nowadays, only bio-engineered skin and negative pressure are recommended for DFU treatment (NICE 2015). Regarding antiseptics, NICE does not contemplate their use as advanced therapeutics. Low-level light therapy and bacteriophage treatment were not considered by NICE, probably due to the lack of reliable studies and the existence of a regulatory gap in the case of bacteriophages.

NICE also considers that the following treatments should not be applied to DFU treatment: autologous platelet-rich plasma gel; regenerative wound matrices; dalteparin, a low–molecular weight heparin (Fragmin; Pharmacia); epidermal growth factor; and transforming growth factor beta (NICE 2015).

Antiseptics

Antiseptics are antimicrobial agents that can be applied on intact skin and some open wounds to eliminate (bactericidal action) or inhibit the multiplication (bacteriostatic action) of bacteria (McDonnell and Russell 1999).

Unlike conventional antibiotics, antiseptics are known for having multiple and unspecific microbial cell targets, including disruption of the bacterial cell membrane (Kramer et al. 2018). For that reason, antiseptics often present a broad antimicrobial spectrum of action and are less susceptible of losing their efficacy due to development of antimicrobial resistance, when compared to antibiotics that generally possess only one specific cell target (Dumville et al. 2017). Antiseptics are widely used in hospitals worldwide to decrease, inhibit, or eliminate pathogenic microorganisms (Hirsch et al. 2010).

A major disadvantage of old generation antiseptics was their toxicity regarding several host cells and tissues, like fibroblasts, keratinocytes, and leucocytes (Wilson et al. 2005). For that reason, antiseptics lost some of their importance for more than a century. With the development of a variety of newer, more efficient and safer antiseptic compounds, along with the spread of antibiotic-resistant microorganisms, wound antiseptics have recovered their role in clinical practice (Dumville et al. 2017; Kramer et al. 2018).

The main antiseptics in use or under consideration to be used in advanced DFU therapeutics include acetic acid, iodine compounds, hexachlorophene, chlorhexidine gluconate, polyhexamethylene biguanide, and octenidine dihydrochloride.

Acetic acid is an antiseptic agent with bactericidal activity against most gram-positive and gram-negative bacteria, including *Pseudomonas aeruginosa*, an important bacterial species associated with DFI (Agrawal et al. 2017; Kavitha et al. 2014). Due to its low price and high availability, acetic acid is frequently used in countries with limited resources for the management of chronic wounds, such as DFU (Agrawal et al. 2017). However, its cytotoxic effects and limited activity against biofilm-based bacteria led to a significant decrease of its clinical use (Dumville et al. 2017; Saad, Khoo, and Halim 2013).

Iodine compounds exhibit a broad microbiocidal activity against protozoa, fungi, yeasts, bacteria, and viruses, but are no longer frequently used due to their high toxicity (Kramer et al. 2018; McDonnell and Russell 1999). Povidone iodine and cadexomer iodine are the exceptions. These antiseptics present reduced local toxicity compared to other iodine products and can be used in wet ulcers and wounds, being indicated for perioperative skin cleansing. Povidone iodine is more effective in infected acute wounds, whereas cadexomer iodine is more efficient in chronic wounds (Murdoch and Lagan, 2013). Cadexomer iodine may also be used in dressings showing a broad-spectrum antimicrobial activity, with decreased rates of bacterial resistance development and contact sensitivity (Richmond, Vivas, and Kirsner 2013). Nevertheless, it is important to refer that povidone iodine and cadexomer iodine should be used with caution in patients with systemic complications, such as renal dysfunction and thyroid disorders (Kramer et al. 2018; Murdoch and Lagan, 2013).

Hexachlorophene is an old generation biguanide with bacteriostatic effect against gram-positive bacteria, including *Staphylococcus* species. Currently, hexachlorophene is no longer recommended for routine application on wounds due to its toxicity to the central nervous system and skin (Dumville et al. 2017).

Chlorhexidine gluconate is a biguanide with a broader spectrum of action, with demonstrated activity against gram-positive bacteria, including *S. aureus*, and gram-negative bacteria, such as *P. aeruginosa*. Additionally, chlorhexidine persistent activity may last up to 6 hours after application and it is indicated as a surgical hand scrub and skin and wound cleanser (Milstone, Passaretti, and Perl 2008). Chlorhexidine use may cause adverse effects hypersensitivity reactions, such as anaphylaxis (Krautheim, Jermann, and Bircher 2004), dermatitis (Osmundsen 1982) and corneal injury (Anders and Wollensak 1997).

Polyhexamethylene biguanide, also known as polyhexanide, is a recent biguanide with a spectrum of action and residual activity equivalent to chlorhexidine (Sibbald, Coutts, and Woo 2011). Its structure, formed by polyhexamethylene monomers, resembles the structure of chlorhexidine, except for the terminal NH-group, which represents a small molecular modification that allows polyhexamethylene to exhibit a similar antiseptic efficacy and a better tolerability when compared to chlorhexidine (Kramer et al. 2018; Sibbald, Coutts, and Woo 2011). Therefore, it is indicated for the management of chronic and infected wounds, including DFU (To et al. 2016).

Recently, octenidine dihydrochloride has emerged as the weapon of choice in the treatment of persistently infected DFU, mainly due to its antimicrobial activity against *P. aeruginosa* and *S. aureus* biofilms (Hubner, Siebert, and Kramer 2010; Junka et al. 2014). Like chlorhexidine and polyhexamethylene, octenidine also displays residual antimicrobial activity (Kramer et al. 2018). *In vitro*, octenidine can stimulate phagocytosis and growth factors production, including the platelet-derived growth factor, supporting its application as an adjuvant therapy in the management of DFU (Hubner, Siebert, and Kramer 2010).

In conclusion, new antiseptics with improved activity are available for the treatment of infected DFU. Their selection should be based on ulcer grade, the characteristics of the infectious microbiota, and type of dressings applied, aiming at avoiding cross-reactivity with certain wound dressings (Hirsch et al. 2010).

Bio-Engineered Skin

Bio-engineered skin was used during the last decades as a new therapeutic method to treat DFU. There are several skin substitute products available in the market (57 in 2012), but only two are premarket approved by the Food and Drug Administration (FDA). The only human- and human/animal-derived products regulated through the premarket approval are an allogeneic bilayered cultured skin equivalent, Apligraf/Graftskin, and a human fibroblast-derived dermal substitute, Dermagraft (Snyder, Sullivan, and Schoelles 2012).

Apligraf and Dermagraft are not indicated to be applied to infected wounds. As they are living cells, their use involves the risk of immune rejection and infection transmission. In fact, the maternal blood of the neonatal donor and the working cell banks must be screened for pathogens, infectious agents, and other contaminants (Wu, Marston, and Armstrong 2010). Unlike human skin, Apligraf does not contain any antigen presenting cells such as Langerhans cells and macrophages, or inflammatory cells such as lymphocytes and other leucocytes, or other tissue structures such as blood vessels or hair follicles (Zaulyanov and Kirsner 2007). As well, Dermagraft does not contain macrophages, lymphocytes, blood vessels, or hair follicles (Wu, Marston, and Armstrong 2010).

Apligraf (Graftskin; Orangogenesis Inc, Canton, MA) was the first allogeneic bilayered cultured skin equivalent approved by the United States FDA in 1998 and 2000 for, respectively, the treatment of full-thickness chronic venous ulcers (with a duration of >1 month) and full-thickness neuropathic DFU (with a duration of >3 weeks) extending through the dermis but without tendon, muscle, joint capsule, or bone exposure (Wu, Marston, and Armstrong 2010; Zaulyanov and Kirsner 2007). It is packed in a sealed heavy-gauge polyethylene bag with a 10% CO_2 atmosphere, and an agarose nutrient medium maintained under a controlled temperature between 20°C and 23°C and must be used within 15 minutes after opening (Wu, Marston, and Armstrong 2010).

Apligraf is developed from the neonatal foreskin, it has an upper epidermal and a lower dermal layer and contains human skin cells and structural proteins that produce all cytokines and growth factors necessary for the healing process. The epidermal layer is composed of human keratinocytes whereas the dermal layer is formed by human fibroblasts in a bovine type I collagen matrix. Human epidermal keratinocytes are prompt to multiply and then to differentiate and replicate the architecture of the human epidermis, forming this way the upper epidermal layer, which acts as a barrier against infection and fluid loss (Veves et al. 2001). Human neonatal dermal fibroblasts are cultured on bovine type I collagen matrix and allowed to stratify. They produce additional matrix proteins, which organized together with the provided structural proteins allow the formation of the lower dermal layer. Fibroblasts and keratinocytes cells that constitute Apligraf appear to present a relatively short life, resisting less than 4 weeks in most patients (Zaulyanov and Kirsner 2007). It costs US$51/cm^2, has a 10-day shelf life and is recommended to be applied weekly (Garfein 2009).

Apligraf provides immediate wound coverage, and it seems to act by filling in the wound with extracellular matrix and by inducing the expression and production of different growth factors and mediators such as interleukin transforming growth factors (TGF-β) and cytokines that contribute to wound healing by three mechanisms: secondary intention, persistent wound closure with underlying healing, and frank graft take (Zaulyanov and Kirsner 2007; De, Reis, and Kerstein 2002; Veves et al. 2001).

A recent study stated that blood flow increased around 72% in the base of five of seven-foot ulcers treated with Apligraft. This result may reflect angiogenesis in the new tissue and/or vasodilatation of existing vessels promoted by the bioengineered skin (Newton et al. 2002).

According to a clinical trial, 56% of DFU treated with Apligraf were totally closed after 12 weeks, compared with 39% of ulcers treated with conventional therapy ($P < 0.05$). The median time required for wound closure was 25 days shorter for DFU treated with Apligraf than with conventional therapy ($P < 0.05$) (Veves et al. 2001).

According to a study using a Markov-based simulation model the treatment with Apligraf plus good wound care led to a 12% reduction in costs during the first year of treatment when compared with good wound care practices alone. In addition, the use of Apligraf increased ulcer-free time and reduced the risk of amputation, counterbalancing the initial costs of the product (Redekop et al. 2003).

Apligraf is susceptible to some antiseptics like the Dakin's solution, povidone-iodine and chlorhexidine; therefore, these should not be used for disinfection prior to Apligraf. Apligraf is recognized as being immunologically inert, showing no clinical evidence of rejection (Zaulyanov and Kirsner 2007).

Dermagraft (Advanced Bio Healing, Inc, La Jolla, CA) was approved by the United States FDA in 2001 for the treatment of chronic and full-thickness DFU (with a duration of >6 weeks) extending through the dermis but without tendon, muscle, joint capsule, or bone exposure. It is packaged with bovine serum and a saline-based cryoprotectant that contains 10% dimethyl sulfoxide (Wu, Marston, and Armstrong 2010).

Dermagraft, as Apligraf, has a dermal component derived from neonatal fibroblasts, but it does not contain an epidermal component or bovine collagen (Garfein 2009). Dermagraft is a cryopreserved human fibroblast-derived dermal substitute, composed of fibroblasts, extracellular matrix, and a bioabsorbable scaffold. It is produced using human dermal fibroblast cells from newborn foreskin tissue that are cultured on top of a bioabsorbable polyglactin mesh scaffold. As the fibroblasts grow and fill the scaffold, they secrete collagen, matrix proteins, growth factors, glycosaminoglycans, and cytokines, generating a three-dimensional, allogeneic, human dermal substitute. Dermagraft contains metabolically active cells that present a nearly parallel alignment of their collagen fibers (Marston 2004). It costs US\$34/cm^2 and has a six-month shelf life (Garfein 2009).

Several studies showed that human fibroblast-derived dermal substitute promotes the healing of chronic ulcers (Hanft and Surprenant 2002; Marston et al. 2003). In one study, 30.0% of patients to whom human fibroblast-derived dermal substitute was applied were able to heal their ulcers, in comparison with 18.3% of control patients (Marston et al. 2003); in another study, 71.4% of the patients to whom human fibroblast-derived dermal substitute was applied were able to heal their ulcers in comparison with 14.3% of control patients (Hanft and Surprenant 2002).

Human fibroblast-derived dermal substitute assists in the restoration of the dermal layer of an ulcer by two different ways: first, it facilitates angiogenesis though the deposition of matrix proteins (Mansbridge 1998); second, it facilitates the patient's own epithelial cells to migrate through the collagen matrix and to close the wound by bouding to growth factors and receptors (Mansbridge et al. 1998).

Dermagraft is safe, and there has been no reported cases of the development of immune response leading to its rejection by an allogeneic host. This may be explained by the fact that human fibroblast-derived dermal substitute is derived from neonatal human tissue that does not develop leukocyte antigen tissue markers, and that especially does not express human leukocyte antigen-DR markers, which are the antigens more frequently responsible for graft loss (Mansbridge et al. 1998; Marston et al. 2003).

According to observational studies and using a Markov model to evaluate the cost-effectiveness of Dermagraft in addition to conventional DFU treatments, the application of Dermagraft allowed an average cost decrease of 37.4% (Langer and Rogowski 2009).

The application of Dermagraft and Apligraf requires rapid identification of nonhealing wounds in patients receiving standard care, proper patient selection based on the type of wound, and proper use of the product (Zaulyanov and Kirsner 2007). A nonhealing wound is defined as a wound that does not adequately respond to conventional, standard therapy within a three- to a four-week period (Cavorsi et al. 2006). Dermagraft and Apligraf should be used in conjunction with standard wound care regimens and in patients that have adequate blood supply to the involved foot (Wu, Marston, and Armstrong 2010). Surgical revascularization, decompression, and wound bed preparation should be performed prior to bioengineering skin application because peripheral ischemia critically affects skin transplantation. The strict control of any signs of infection should be implemented after skin allografts application (Yazdanpanah, Nasiri, and Adarvish 2015). They are both contraindicated for use on clinically infected wounds or ulcers with sinus tracts and in patients with known hypersensitivity to bovine products (Wu, Marston, and Armstrong 2010).

Chronic inflammation and impaired angiogenesis are the backbones of DFU recurrence. Inefficient angiogenesis prolongs ulceration and increases the probability of amputation. According to Wildgerow (Wildgerow 2014), current bioengineered skin therapies do not adequately target vasculogenesis. The author proposes that newer designs of bioengineered skin may give rise to a new generation of products more focused on promoting collagen production, cellular proliferation, and particularly vasculogenesis while controlling infection.

According to NICE, dermal or skin substitutes should be used as a complement to standard care in DFU treatment only when healing does not progress (Table 1) (NICE 2015).

Negative Pressure Wound Therapy

Negative Pressure Wound Therapy (NPWT) includes a set of medical procedures used to seal wounds by creating a near airtight setting in which a sub-atmospheric pressure is applied (Banwell and Teot 2003; Nain et al. 2011; Panayi, Leavitt, and Orgill 2017). In a NPWT setting, the wound is usually filled with a porous material like gauze or open-pore sponge, facilitating pressure transmission between the wound and a drainage tube connected to a vacuum pump. The wound is sealed with an adhesive drape allowing the generation of negative pressures typically between -50 and -150mm Hg (Huang et al. 2014; Panayi, Leavitt, and Orgill 2017), being -125mm Hg the clinical standard pressure generally applied (Borgquist, Ingemansson, and Malmsjo 2010).

NPWT has been used as a complementary treatment in several human diseases, such as acute, chronic and postsurgical wounds, open fractures, grafts and flaps, pressure ulcers and particularly DFU (Apelqvist et al. 2017; Hasan, Teo, and Nather 2015). Regarding DFU patients, this therapeutic procedure has been acknowledged for more than two decades, persisting nowadays as one of the most commonly used complementary approaches in patients with this disease (Borys et al. 2019a).

NPWT was firstly used in wound management due to its efficacy in the collection of wound exudate, contributing for decreasing local edema and keeping wounds clean, therefore reducing the frequency of dressing changes and preventing bacterial colonization (Borys et al. 2019a; Liu et al. 2018; Nain et al. 2011; Schintler 2012). Moreover, other beneficial effects occurring both macroscopically and at the cellular level have been described. In addition to exudate removal, it has been observed that NPWT directly increases perfusion and leads to wound contraction or macro deformation due to the application of mechanical forces to the wound, therefore approaching wound edges and promoting epithelialization (Borys et al. 2019a; Nain et al. 2011; Schintler 2012). There are also alterations at the cellular level or micro deformations that have been shown to promote angiogenesis and reduce the activity of matrix metalloproteinases. These changes are important to neovascularization, improving blood flow, extracellular matrix remodeling and generation of granulation tissue, all essential for proper wound healing (Gary Sibbald and Woo 2008; Greene et al. 2006; Ravanti and Kahari 2000).

NPWT may also promote the alteration of the wound microenvironment leading to the reduction of the local inflammatory status (Wang et al. 2017; Wang et al. 2019). NPWTs' anti-inflammatory effect is a direct result of the decrease in the synthesis of pro-inflammatory enzymes and cytokines, such as IL-6, TNF-α, and iNOS, following IkB-α inhibition, which prevents the activation of NF-κB during ulcer healing (Wang et al. 2017; Wang et al. 2019). It has also been reported that NPWT mediates differential gene expression of several key growth factors, such as vascular endothelial growth factor and fibroblast growth factor 2 while reducing the expression of inflammatory cytokines (Borys et al. 2019b; Tanaka et al. 2016; Wang et al. 2017). This anti-inflammatory effect contributes considerably to the success of DFU treatment by increasing wound healing rate, decreasing healing time and reducing the amputation risk (Wang et al. 2017).

Despite NPWT benefits, some potentially negative effects have also been described. These include wound maceration, retention of dressings, pain and wound infection (Dumville et al. 2013; Liu et al. 2018). NPWT devices can also interfere with mobility and may cause sleep problems in some patients (Dumville et al. 2013). The implementation of more comprehensive studies on adverse events (e.g., pain and infection) and quality of life of these patients, will be valuable for a broader evaluation of the procedure.

Moreover, systematic reviews of several clinical studies supporting the use of the technique identified some methodological flaws, making it difficult to evaluate the significance of the measured outcomes such as granulation tissue formation rate, proportion of patients with complete wound healing or amputation rates in DFU patients treated with this technique. Therefore, to date, it was not possible to establish a clear superiority of NPWT over any other dressing type (Wynn 2019).

Nevertheless, NPWT should be considered a generally safe treatment for DFU patients (Armstrong and Lavery 2005; Blume et al. 2008; Sepúlveda et al. 2009), without significant association with adverse events (Nain et al. 2011). NPWT is recommended by NICE guidelines for the treatment of DFU, to be considered following surgical debridement (Table 1) (NICE 2015). Also, international guidelines point NPWT as an important adjuvant therapy for DFU, which use is expected to increase after further and solid evidence of its potential to improve DFU outcome (Apelqvist et al. 2017; Game et al. 2016).

Electrical Stimulation

Electrical Stimulation (ES) is a therapeutic procedure that consists in the delivery of an external low electrical current through an equipment comprising two or more electrodes with opposite charges, positioned on the surface of tissues or wounds under medical treatment, aiming to accelerate the healing process (Thakral et al. 2013). The current delivered by the electrodes may be of different types (e.g., direct or pulsed current) and its duration, frequency or amplitude can also vary. Usually, the current delivered is unbalanced, as observed for high-voltage pulsed current, promoting the accumulation of a small charge beneath the electrodes (Houghton 2017; Sari et al. 2017).

The application of therapeutic ES is based on the knowledge that the epidermis of intact skin exhibits a physiological electrical potential resulting from the uneven distribution of ions along the tissue (Foulds and Barker 1983) and that an eventual damage of the epidermis, such as wound development, causes a change in the electrical potential (Braddock, Campbell, and Zuder 1999). That change results in the establishment of a low current flux between the epidermis and underlying tissues (Jaffe and Vanable 1984; Nuccitelli et al. 2008) that together with other mechanisms, such as chemotaxis and mediation of cell migration, have been shown to contribute to wound healing (Thakral et al. 2013; Zhao 2009; Zhao et al. 2006).

Given the recognized role of endogenous electrical fields in wound healing, it has been proposed more than 50 years ago that exogenous ES could be used in therapeutic protocols (Assimacopoulos 1968; Braddock, Campbell, and Zuder 1999). Initial studies using cell culture and animals (Torkaman 2014) and several other studies in humans have showed the beneficial effects of ES on accelerating the healing of both acute and chronic wounds (Adunsky and Ohry 2005; Feedar, Kloth, and Gentzkow 1991; Houghton et al. 2010; Machado et al. 2016), including DFU (Lundeberg, Eriksson, and Malm 1992; Sari et al. 2017).

The mechanisms underlying the effects of electrical current on wound healing are not completely understood. It is believed that ES imitates the natural electrical current that occurs in the wound healing process (Thakral et al. 2013). It was demonstrated that the application of an electrical field is able to stimulate the migration of different types of cells, such as epithelial cells, macrophages, mast cells, and granulocytes, along a voltage gradient (Zhao 2009). Specifically, direct current is able to attract granulocytes towards the cathode and guide these cells towards the wound exudate, facilitating wound debridement (Braddock, Campbell, and Zuder 1999).

Moreover, several studies also showed that ES is able to improve blood flow at wound site through the promotion of angiogenesis and up-regulating the expression of angiogenic markers such as Vascular Endothelial Growth Factor A (VEGF-A) and Placental Growth Factor, that persist for several days after the application of ES (Ud-Din et al. 2015). This effect is particularly interesting given the important role of angiogenesis and neo-vascularization on wound healing (Greaves et al. 2013; Tonnesen, Feng, and Clark 2000).

It has also been shown that ES promotes the synthesis of collagen and migration of keratinocytes in ischemic DFU through the release of vascular growth factors such as VEGF and hypoxia-inducible factor 1-α (Asadi et al. 2017; Wirsing et al. 2015). This outcome is relevant given the importance of collagen synthesis regulation in the transition from provisional wound matrix to a collagenous scar and effective wound closure (Clark 1998; Singer and Clark 1999). It has also been shown that ES may also reduce pain associated with wound healing (Solis et al. 2011).

Several studies have reported a reduction in inflammation following the application of ES (Odell and Sorgnard 2008; Sari et al. 2017; Sebastian et al. 2011). This effect may be due to the ability of ES to direct the migration of excessive neutrophils, monocytes, and macrophages away from the site of injury. ES may also reduce inflammation by decreasing the number of CD3+ cells at the wound site (Sebastian et al. 2011).

Results from some well-designed randomized clinical trials and high-quality systematic reviews consistently support the fact that ES can improve wound size reduction or wound closure, providing strong support for the use of ES on various types of chronic wounds (Houghton 2017). However, several randomized controlled trials showed that ES has no effect on wound healing outcome (Everett and Mathioudakis 2018; Game et al. 2016b).

In conclusion, there is no consensus regarding the detailed effects of ES on wound healing, and its use is not recommended (NICE 2015). More well-designed studies with a higher number of patients are needed before ES can be extensively recommended as a treatment for DFU.

Recombinant Human Platelet-Derived Growth Factor

Wound healing is a complex coordinated process of biological and molecular events that include the production of inflammatory mediators, growth factors, cytokines, the remodeling of extracellular matrix and the involvement of several cell types (Han and Ceilley 2017; Velnar, Bailey, and Smrkolj 2009). Throughout this process, a variety of cellular responses occur, including the recruitment and activation of platelets and the onset of the coagulation cascade (Golebiewska and Poole 2015). At the wound site, platelets release cytokine-loaded granules, including alpha platelet granules, rich in growth factors such as the Platelet Derived Growth Factor (PDGF) (Eppley, Woodell, and Higgins 2004; Golebiewska and Poole 2015; Grazul-Bilska et al. 2003; Werner and Grose 2003).

As previously mentioned, patients with diabetes are likely to develop several complications including impaired wound healing (Falanga 2005) and DFU, that have a tendency to chronicity (Armstrong, Boulton, and Bus 2017; Ince, Game, and Jeffcoate 2007). Chronic foot ulcers are often stalled in the inflammatory phase, presenting an accumulation of advanced glycation end-products, enhanced aldose reductase activity, increased protein kinase C activity, increased hexosamine pathway flux, and over-stimulation of the polyol pathway, all contributing to poor healing (Gary Sibbald and Woo 2008). Moreover, hyperglycemia *per se* has a negative effect on neutrophil function affecting the wound healing cascade, for instance, by altering the production of enzymes such as elastases and metalloproteinases (Menke et al. 2007). These pathological alterations lead to the degradation of the extracellular matrix, impaired formation of granulation tissue and altered expression of growth factors required for appropriate healing, including a decreased expression of PDGF (Andrae, Gallini, and Betsholtz 2008; Blakytny and Jude 2009; Grazul-Bilska et al. 2003).

The PDGF acts early in the wound-healing cascade modulating chemotaxis and activation of macrophages, monocytes, and neutrophils, therefore modifying the inflammatory response (Deuel et al. 1982; Foster et al. 2009; Martí-Carvajal et al. 2015; Rozman and Bolta 2007; Tzeng et al. 1985). PDGF also stimulates the mitogenesis in fibroblasts and in a variety of mesenchymal-derived cells, promoting angiogenesis and formation of granulation tissue (Eppley, Woodell, and Higgins 2004; Frechette, Martineau, and Gagnon 2005; Pierce et al. 1995; Siegbahn et al. 1990).

Given the effects of PDGF in the initiation and modulation of wound healing, it has been studied as a therapeutic option for the treatment of ulcers, including in diabetic patients (Bennett et al. 2003; del Pino-Sedeno et al. 2019; Martí-Carvajal et al. 2015; Piccin et al. 2017; Shan et al. 2013; Steed et al. 2006). Accordingly, therapeutic approaches using PDGF have been recognized as promising complementary therapies for nonhealing DFU (Khashim et al. 2019).

A recombinant form of human PDGF (rhPDGF) was developed and it has been used in the treatment of DFU with reported success (Margolis et al. 2005; Robson et al. 2005; Robson et al. 1992; Rangaswamy, Rubby, and Prasanth 2016; Steed and The Diabetic Ulcer Study Group 1995). The biological activity of rhPDGF was shown to be similar to the endogenous PDGF, specifically regarding chemotactic recruitment and proliferation of cells involved in wound repair (Nagai and Embil 2002). A commercial rhPDGF (rhPDGF-BB/Becaplermin) was approved by the FDA for topical applications (Hollinger et al. 2008; LeGrand 1998; Wieman, Smiell, and Su 1998). It has been shown to increase the thickness of the granulation tissue in the wound, fibroblast proliferation, collagen production and neovascularization (Robson et al. 2005; Pierce et al. 1994). Becaplermin was already evaluated through extensive animal and human studies, which demonstrated its efficacy as a therapy for DFU when used in combination with standard wound healing practices (Nagai and Embil 2002; Sridharan and Sivaramakrishnan 2018). Moreover, it has been shown that becaplermin contributes for an increased number of diabetic patients with complete foot ulcers healing when compared with those to whom a placebo was administered, decreasing amputation risk and providing better outcomes at a lower cost (Martí-Carvajal et al. 2015; Waycaster, Gilligan, and Motley 2016).

Despite the beneficial effects, the use of PDGF may carry some risks. For instance, PDGF was associated with conditions characterized by excessive cell proliferation, such as fibrotic diseases and atherosclerosis (Bonner 2004; He et al. 2015). Additionally, PDGF stimulates the proliferation of cancer-associated fibroblasts and promotes angiogenesis, suggesting an association with tumor progression (Heldin, Lennartsson, and Westermark 2018). Furthermore, the use of rhPDGF in high dosage (3 or more tubes of becaplermin) was associated with an increase in cancer related mortality (Papanas and Maltezos 2010). In contrast, other studies reported that topical applications of this growth factor are safe and well tolerated (Edmonds et al. 2000; Perry et al. 2002; Prompers et al. 2007; Wieman, Smiell, and Su 1998) and do not increase the risk of cancer development or related mortality (Ziyadeh et al. 2011).

Consequently, despite the promising results of rhPDGF therapeutic use in DFU, more studies are required to clarify its safety. According to NICE, rhPDGF should not be used as a complementary treatment for in-hospital patients, unless as part of a clinical trial (NICE 2015). Potential risks need to be carefully assessed through large randomized clinical trials before generalized use can be recommended.

Hyperbaric Oxygen Therapy

Hyperbaric oxygen therapy (HBOT) has been used as a novel adjuvant treatment for chronic DFU. In HBOT, patients are placed in a hyperbaric chamber and exposed to 100% oxygen at pressures higher than the normal atmospheric pressure at sea level (Bakker 2000; Strauss 2005).

Wound healing is a complex mechanism that occurs through various phases and oxygen is an essential component of this process. The role of oxygen in wound repair is well established and tissue regeneration is limited by its availability at the cellular level (Thackham, McElwain, and Long 2008). An elevated tissue oxygen tension supports the increased energy demand by regeneration tissues and stimulates the presence of growth factors, activation, and replication of fibroblasts, mobility of macrophages, ingrowth of granulation tissue and angiogenesis mechanisms, while decreasing the presence of inflammatory cytokines on wound areas (Chen et al. 2007). Moreover, derivatives of oxygen, such as reactive oxygen species, also play a role in wound regeneration through regulation of cell proliferation, neovascularization, and synthesis of extracellular matrix (Dunnill et al. 2017). In addition, considering that some antibiotics, such as aminoglycosides, require the presence of oxygen to function, an elevated tension of oxygen is also important for promoting antibiotics action (Hermann 2007).

Based on the concept that increasing the oxygen levels on wound areas may improve tissue regeneration and wound healing, HBOT is frequently used in clinical practice (Lipsky and Berendt 2010). In HBOT, a patient enters a hyperbaric chamber that can be single- or multi-occupant and 100% oxygen is administered while the environmental pressure is gradually increased to 2 to 3 atmospheric pressure, increasing the oxygen concentration in blood and tissues by up to 20-fold (Bakker 2000; Strauss 2005). The majority of HBOT protocols for treating refractory DFU require the patient to stay inside the hyperbaric chamber for 90 minutes during 20 to 30 treatments, contrasting with standard wound care that usually involves fewer visits to clinical units (Fedorko et al. 2016; Lipsky and Berendt 2010).

Some studies regarding the therapeutic effect of HBOT on diabetic patients, support the use of this therapy as a complement to conventional DFU treatments to improve ulcer healing and decrease the amputation rates associated with this disease (Abidia et al. 2003; Chen et al. 2010; Duzgun et al. 2008; Faglia et al. 1996; Heyneman and Lawless-Liday 2002; Kessler et al. 2003). Additionally, adverse effects following HBOT, such as ear discomfort, nausea, and blurred vision, are usually temporary and easily resolved, with most patients experiencing no negative effects (Plafki et al. 2000; Wu 2018).

Nonetheless, the application of HBOT as an adjuvant DFU treatment has been controversial. Some clinical trials and systematic reviews on the effectiveness of HBOT suggested conflicting evidence (Lipsky and Berendt 2010; Lipsky et al. 2016). Most studies on HBOT were hampered by small sample size, clinical heterogeneity in terms of ulcer characteristics and therapeutic protocols, inadequate evaluation of external conditions relevant to wound healing, potential bias regarding outcome evaluation and other methodological problems that restrained the ability to establish a definitive recommendation to the usefulness of HBOT as routine treatment of chronic DFU (Duzgun et al. 2008; Faglia et al. 1996; Kessler et al. 2003; Wunderlich, Peters, and Lavery 2000).

Three recent randomized and placebo-controlled clinical trials on the efficacy of HBOT in DFU patients reported that HBOT presented no statistically significant advantage on improving wound healing and decreasing amputation rates compared with standard wound care alone (Fedorko et al. 2016; Zhao et al. 2017; Santema et al. 2018), and therefore it is not recommended as an adjuvant treatment for in-hospital patients (NICE 2015).

Considering that HBOT requires significant patient compliance, time and financial commitment, further studies are needed, mainly to better understand which patients are more likely to benefit from HBOT, decide the appropriate time to initiate this therapy, the optimal duration of treatment, and to determine which treatment protocols are most adequate (Lipsky and Berendt 2010). In conclusion, properly designed clinical trials focusing on large populations are required in order to definitely establish the relevance of this therapy in DFU treatment.

Granulocyte-Colony Stimulating Factor

The granulocyte-colony stimulating factor (G-CSF) is an endogenous hematopoietic growth factor, a cytokine, that induces terminal differentiation and release of neutrophils from the bone marrow, which are often impaired in people with diabetes (Gough et al. 1997). It specifically enhances neutrophil functions by stimulating the growth of both normal and defective neutrophils in people with diabetes (Nelson et al. 2000; Sato et al. 1997), including those with DFI (Peck et al. 2001), playing a central role in the host response to infection (Dale et al. 1995). It also has immunomodulatory and antibiotic-enhancing functions contributing to the control of infectious diseases (Hartung 1999). It is usually administered via injection (subcutaneously, intramuscularly or intravenously), being shown that local administration is more effective promoting wound healing than systemic administration (Shen 2016).

G-CSF is broadly used after bone marrow transplant or suppression after cancer chemotherapy; to reduce incidence and sequelae of neutropenia (low neutrophil count) in patients with conditions like myelodysplastic disorders; to treat infectious diseases by enhancing inflammatory response even if the host has a normal number of neutrophils and normal bone marrow (de Lalla, Nicolin, and Lazzarini 2000; Murata 2003; Root and Dale 1999). It has been reported that G-CSF also contributes to tissue repair in post-myocardial infarction by mobilizing neutrophils and macrophages (Minatoguchi et al. 2004), acting directly on cardiomyocytes and monocytes through the G-CSF receptor (Li et al. 2007).

G-CSF has also been used in DFU treatment along with stem cell therapy (Lopes et al. 2018). In a study with a total of 127 patients with DFU, different doses of G-CSF were administered to these individuals for hematopoietic stem cells mobilization, after which the stem cell suspension was extracted and injected into the ischemic lower extremities along the blood vessels. The authors found that administration of G-CSF significantly increased the blood supply of the lower extremities in DFU patients, relieving pain and cold sensation in the affected limb and gradually promoting ulcer healing (Xu and Liang 2016).

Recently, a comprehensive meta-analysis survey aiming to establish the effects of G-CSF use as a complementary therapy in DFU patients has evaluated main databases and included five trials comprising 167 patients. The authors concluded that the administration of G-CSF preparations, independently of the dose and treatment duration, was associated with a significantly reduced number of lower extremity surgical interventions, including amputation, but did not significantly affect infection development or wound healing. Moreover, treatment reduced the duration of hospitalization but did not significantly affect the duration of systemic antibiotic therapy (Cruciani 2013).

In 2012, the Infectious Diseases Society of America stated that the available data on the efficacy of G-CSF administration to patients with DFU does not support the routine use of G-CSF treatment (Lipsky et al. 2012). Similarly, NICE stated that G-CSF should not be used as a complementary treatment for in-hospital patients (NICE 2015). Although other studies showed the significant efficacy of G-CSF treatment (Xu and

Liang 2016), its use is not recommended given the costs associated and the lack of significant contribution for healing and infections treatment, as described in most studies (Cruciani 2013).

Low-Level Light Therapy

Low-level light therapy (LLLT), also known as low-level laser therapy, can be defined as the application of direct low-level light energy to the surface of the body, in order to stimulate the molecules and atoms of skin cells without causing a significant increase in tissue temperature (Basford 1995; Karu 1989).

Light penetration depth in human tissues can be directly related to light wavelengths (Avci et al. 2013; Barum et al. 2007). Ultraviolet light (150-380 nm) barely penetrates more than 0.1 mm within tissues, whereas violet-deep blue (390-470 nm), blue-green (475-545 nm) and yellow-orange (545-600 nm) lights can penetrate approximately 0.3, 0.3-0.5 and 0.5-1.0 mm, respectively, reaching the epidermis and dermis. Red (600-650 nm) and near-infrared (650-950 nm) lights penetrate further within tissues, around 1.0-2.0 and 2.0-3.0 mm, respectively, reaching the deepest skin layer, the hypodermis. On the other hand, higher wavelengths, namely the infrared spectrum (>950 nm) are associated with smaller penetration depth, of <1 mm (Avci et al. 2013). For that reason, wavelengths in the range of 390-600 nm are used in the treatment of superficial tissues diseases, whereas wavelengths in the range of 600-950 nm, with an ability to further penetrate within tissues, are preferred for the treatment of deeper tissues diseases (Barolet 2008). In LLLT, tissues are exposed to wavelengths between 650 nm and 900 nm, approximately, and light can be applied in continuous or pulsed waves. Also, the fluences (0.04-50 J/cm^2) and power densities (25-200 mW/cm^2) used are generally low (AlGhamdi, Kumar, and Moussa 2012; Kazemi-Khoo 2006).

The photobiostimulatory effects of LLLT were discovered in the late 1960s. However, only recently LLLT has been regularly used as adjuvant therapy for skin healing and repair (Kazemi-Khoo 2006). LLLT is known for stimulating a variety of cellular processes, contributing for the reduction of inflammation and the increase of cell proliferation and tissue regeneration (Barolet 2008; Chung et al. 2012; Karu and Kolyakov 2005; Peplow et al. 2011).

The mechanism of action of LLLT is not fully understood yet. However, it has been suggested that the absorption of red and near-infrared light by mitochondrial chromophores, particularly cytochrome c oxidase, induces a cascade of events leading to enzymes activation, electron transportation and adenosine triphosphate production (Karu and Kolyakov 2005; Karu, Pyatibrat, and Kalendo 2004). Ultimately, this process changes the redox state of cells and is responsible for the activation of several intracellular signaling pathways, resulting in a broad range of effects at the molecular, cellular and tissue levels (Karu and Kolyakov 2005; Liu et al. 2005; Peplow et al. 2011).

The promising properties of LLLT regarding wound repair boosted its use as an adjuvant treatment for DFU. The application of low-energy light radiation on ulcer areas has a stimulating effect on migration and proliferation of fibroblasts, skin reepithelization, connective tissue repair and blood microcirculation (Houreld and Abrahamse 2010; Litscher 2012; Schindl et al. 1998). *In vitro* studies using cell cultures gave evidence on the ability of LLLT to reduce wound inflammation via inhibition of prostaglandins and cytokines action (Safavi et al. 2008; Shimizu et al. 1995). Moreover, the induction of reactive oxygen species confers LLLT a direct antibacterial effect, enhancing its potential contribution to infected DFU healing (Lipovsky et al. 2010).

Based on the positive results obtained, clinical trials also encourage the use of LLLT in the treatment of DFU. In a randomized, placebo-controlled, double-blinded clinical trial involving 14 patients with 23 chronic diabetic ulcers, Minatel et al. (2009) reported that the group treated with LLLT (660-890 nm, $3J/cm^2$) presented more granulation tissue and faster healing rates, compared to control group. Studies performed by Saltmarch (2008), Landau et al. (2011), Kaviani et al. (2011) and Kajagar et al. (2012) sustained the results obtained by Minatel et al. (2009) and described a significant reduction of ulcer size and wound closure time in the LLLT group.

Recently, a clinical trial conducted by Priyadarshini, Babu, and Thariq (2018) explored the effects of phototherapy regarding infection control, showing that patients exposed to LLLT presented a reduced rate of culture-positive swabs after 15 days of treatment, compared to control group (Priyadarshini, Babu, and Thariq 2018).

A systematic review and meta-analysis of several randomized controlled trials reported that LLLT has a significant potential to become a portable, low invasive, easy-to-use technique for DFU treatment (Li et al. 2018; Tchanque-Fossuo et al. 2016). LLLT is effective in promoting granulation, reducing ulcer size and improving healing, being cost-effective, especially for superficial and deep ulcers with no bone involvement or abscess (Li et al. 2018).

In summary, numerous clinical trials report the use of LLLT as an effective tool against DFU. However, additional studies with comparable laser parameters, larger sample sizes and longer follow-up periods are required to validate the use of LLLT (Li et al. 2018; Tchanque-Fossuo et al. 2016). More studies are also required to determine which dosimetry parameters (wavelength, power density, energy, polarization, pulse structure, light fluence, irradiation time and administration protocol) provide the best results regarding DFU healing (Avci et al. 2013; Beckmann, Meyer-Hamme, and Schroder 2014).

Bacteriophage Therapy

Bacteriophages, or phages, were first described at the beginning of the '90s by two microbiologists, Felix Twort in 1915 and Felix d'Hérelle in 1917 (Wittebole, De Roock, and Opal 2014). Phages are viruses that present a DNA or RNA genome enclosed within a protein coat, which specifically infect bacteria. They have an ubiquitary distribution, being considered the most predominant organism on Earth (Sulakvelidze 2011).

According to the International Committee for Taxonomy of Viruses, phages are classified in 14 families, with the majority being included in the order *Caudovirales*. Phages from this order present a genome formed by DNA, a regular and symmetric capsid head and a symmetric helical DNA injection tail. This tail can be long and contractile, as observed in phages from the *Myoviridae* family, long and non-contractile, as observed in members from the *Syphoviridae* family, or short, as observed in the *Podoviridae* family (Ackermann, 2009; Taha et al. 2018).

Bacteriophages are considered to be obligatory parasites that can present two different replication cycles, lytic and lysogenic, depending on the degree of genetic interaction with the genetic material of the bacterial host (Burrowes et al. 2011). After infecting bacterial cells, lytic phages immediately start to use the bacterial cell mechanisms to replicate the phage genome and synthesize capsid and tail proteins, in order to produce progeny phages. After packing the new genome molecules into progeny phage particles, these are released through bacterial lysis, with the whole cycle occurring within minutes to hours. On another end, after infecting the bacterial cells, temperate phages may enter a lysogenic cycle, in which the phage genome is integrated into the bacterial chromosome, forming a prophage. Prophages can persist integrated into the bacterial chromosome, being replicated together with the bacterial DNA and transmitted during bacteria multiplication to the resulting daughter cells, until phage genes are activated by environmental factors and a lytic cycle is initiated (Burrowes et al. 2011). The lysogenic cycle may promote gene transfer and consequent dissemination of toxin, virulence and antibiotic resistance genes between bacterial species, which represents a selective advantage for the bacterial host (Wittebole, De Roock, and Opal 2014). Finally, some phages can also present pseudolysogeny, an unstable state which occurs under nutrient-deprived conditions, in which bacterial cells do not perform DNA replication or protein synthesis, and as such phages are also not able to develop a lytic cycle or become prophages (Feiner et al. 2015).

Soon after the discovery of bacteriophages, these organisms began to be applied as therapeutic agents for the control of bacterial infections. In fact, bacteriophage therapy was first used in 1921 by Bruynoghe and

Maisin for the treatment of *S. aureus* skin infections (Wittebole, De Roock, and Opal 2014), but the interest in phage-based therapeutic protocols declined in the 1930s after the discovery and generalized use of antibiotics. By then, the application of bacteriophage therapy declined in western countries, but it remained as an option within the Soviet Union and Eastern Europe, especially in Poland and Georgia (Fish et al. 2018; Lu and Collins 2007; Morozova, Vlassov, and Tikunova 2018). Recently, due to the global dissemination of antibiotic-resistant strains and increased mortality rates due to antibiotic-resistant infections and the lack of effective novel antibiotics in the pipeline, bacteriophage therapy is once again being considered as a valid therapeutic option, and research in this area continues to increase (Abedon et al. 2011; Fish et al. 2018; Knezevic and Petrovic 2008; Morozova, Vlassov, and Tikunova 2018; Smith, Huggins, and Shaw 1987).

Bacteriophage therapy presents several advantages. Due to phage specificity, the inhibitory action of most phages is focused on one single bacterial species or strain, which allows the maintenance of the commensal microbiome and avoidance of the collateral dysbiosis associated with antibiotic therapy (Chen and Novick 2009). Another advantage is that phages only replicate at the site of infection where the target bacteria are present, assuring their safe use and absence of side effects, even if they are administered through a systemic route (Haq et al. 2012). Also, *in situ* replication prompts the increase in phage numbers, which allows avoiding the administration of high concentrations of phages to the site of infection, as required in antibiotherapy (Burrowes et al. 2011). Furthermore, as antibiotics and phage resistance are usually not related, antibiotic-resistant strains can be susceptible to phages. Finally, phage production is simple and cost-effective, with phages being easily manipulated through several techniques (Haq et al. 2012; Wittebole, De Roock, and Opal 2014).

Despite all these advantages, bacteriophage therapy also presents some problems. First, the maintenance of the lytic cycle *in vivo* depends on host factors, particularly on infection temperature (Haq et al. 2012); as such, under particular conditions lytic phages may be able to enter into a temperate cycle, which can have serious consequences, including the dissemination of bacterial virulence determinants (Ghannad and Mohammadi 2012). For this reason, bacteriophage therapy should only be based on the use of lytic phages, and the application of temperate bacteriophages must be prohibited. Also, the extensive lysis of high concentrations of Gram-negative species may lead to endotoxic shock due to the massive release of bacterial endotoxins, as previously described for some bactericidal antibiotics (Rac, Greer, and Wendel 2010). Another concern is the elimination of these viruses from the systemic circulation by both humoral and innate immunity mechanisms, which may impair their efficacy in the case of extended or repeated administration protocols (Clark and March 2006; Dabrowska et al. 2005). Finally, bacterial resistance to phages has already been described. In fact, bacteria have developed several adaptive mechanisms aiming at avoiding phages action (Drulis-Kawa et al. 2012).

The most frequent resistance mechanism is the modification/loss of bacterial receptors, preventing phage adsorption to the bacterial surface and thus impairing the subsequent formation of virus progeny. This can also be achieved through the production of extracellular matrix or release of competitive inhibitors, rendering receptors unavailable to phages (Labrie, Samson, and Moineau 2010). Bacteria can also express several systems that promote the degradation of phage DNA, such as the Restriction-Modification defense system and the Clustered Regularly Interspaced Short Palindromic Repeats (Makarova et al. 2011). These systems can interrupt phage development, replication and progeny release, leading to an abortive infection in which host defense mechanisms promote cell death, thereby preventing the dissemination of infective phages (Stern and Sorek 2011). Finally, bacteria may express Superinfection Exclusion Systems, constituted by proteins that impair the entrance of phage DNA in the host cells, therefore conferring resistance against specific phages (Labrie, Samson, and Moineau 2010). Nevertheless, despite all these mechanisms, the *in vivo* frequency of phage-resistant bacterial strains is reported as low.

In spite of the increasing number of studies focusing on bacteriophage therapy, to date only a few large-scale clinical studies aiming at demonstrating phage safety and efficacy as therapeutic agents were approved by the FDA and the European Medicines Agency (Wittebole, De Roock, and Opal 2014), and, to our knowledge, no phage preparation has been approved for commercialization yet. To date, the most comprehensive records of phage administration for the treatment of human infections were the ones described in the several studies conducted by Slopek and collaborators (Slopek et al. 1983a, 1983b, 1984, 1985a, 1985b, 1985c, 1987), in which oral phages and bacteriophage-soaked compresses were applied in the treatment of localized infections in 550 patients, with a success rate of approximately 92%. In 2009, a first Phase I randomized controlled trial was performed in the United States, aiming at evaluating the consequences of the application of a phage cocktail directed against *Escherichia coli*, *S. aureus* and *P. aeruginosa* to 42 patients with chronic venous leg ulcers. In this trial, bacteriophage therapy was proven to be safe and effective for the management of infected wounds, but before the approval of this cocktail for commercialization, a complementary Phase II trial is necessary, since the posology used in the Phase I study was not in agreement with the available data on bacteriophage pharmacokinetics (Rhoads et al. 2009). More recently, the Phagoburn project, financed by the European Commission under the 7th Framework Program for Research and Development between June 2013 and February 2017, performed the evaluation of the potential of a bacteriophage cocktail for treating burn wounds infected with *E. coli* and *P. aeruginosa*, and included a Phase I-II clinical trial (www.phagoburn.eu).

In fact, infected chronic wounds represent one of the best models for the application of bacteriophage therapy. Among them, DFI are good targets for phage administration, since some intrinsic adverse characteristics, including poor vascularization and the presence of a diverse array of resistant and biofilm-producing strains, render them very recalcitrant to antibiotics action (Mendes et al. 2012; Mendes et al. 2014; Morozova, Vlassov, and Tikunova 2018; Mottola et al. 2016a, 2016b, 2016c). Research aiming at the application of bacteriophage therapy for DFI treatment has been developed in both Europe and the United States (Mendes et al. 2014; Fish et al. 2018; Taha et al. 2018), but an established treatment protocol is still not available in the western world. In a study led by a Portuguese biotech company, Technophage, phage cocktails for the treatment of DFI associated with *S. aureus*, *P. aeruginosa* and *Acinetobacter baumannii* were developed and characterized. Results were very promising, and in 2014, FDA has authorized the development of clinical trials using TP-102, one of the developed bacteriophage cocktails (Mendes et al. 2014).

Finally, it is important to refer that, specific guidelines and standardized protocols aiming at evaluating the safety and efficacy of bacteriophage therapy are required, as regulations from individual countries can be very different. In fact, phages and bacteriophage therapy are not classified into a single category, being considered as biological human medicinal products (Parracho et al. 2012). The currently available regulation for such products establishes the performance of clinical trials and the submission of a complete product dossier in accordance with Directive 2001/83/EG (Huys et al. 2013). To address these issues, a European organization was created for the evaluation of research and clinical trials using bacteriophage therapy, the Phages for Human Applications Group Europe (P.H.A.G.E.) (P.H.A.G.E. 2009).

CONCLUSION

Advanced DFU therapies are important to promote DFU healing in diabetic patients with recalcitrant ulcers, avoiding detrimental consequences such as amputation and improving life quality (Ragnarson and Apelqvist 2004). The combination of some of these therapies with conventional therapeutic protocols has a superior healing effect in comparison with the singular application of the last (Richmond, Vivas, and Kirsner 2013).

Advanced therapies should be considered for recalcitrant diabetic ulcers with low or no response to conventional treatments over a period of 2 weeks (Mulder, Tenenhaus, and D'Souza 2014) or 4 weeks (Richmond, Vivas, and Kirsner 2013), considering the overall health status of the diabetic patient and healing progression. Good practice recommendations and a multidisciplinary team working together, including health and social care providers and commissioners, is needed to an effective outcome. The costs associated with the implementation of advanced therapies and their effectiveness should also be considered (Mulder, Tenenhaus, and D'Souza 2014). Efficient and cost-effective therapies should contribute for the decrease of the overall economic burden associated with DM (WHO 2016; Yazdanpanah, Nasiri, and Adarvish 2015) which, according to estimates, will affect almost US$2 trillion individuals worldwide by 2030 (Bloom et al. 2011).

Among the developed advanced DFU therapies are novel antiseptics. Novel and improved topical antimicrobial therapy has been used on DFU, either to prevent infection or as a treatment for clinically infected wounds (Dumville et al. 2017). They may be used as a perioperative skin cleansing or soaked dressings (Hirsch et al. 2010). In infected foot ulcers antiseptics administration may be preferable to systemic antibiotherapy due to their broad-spectrum antimicrobial activity and decreased rates of bacterial resistance (Dumville et al. 2017; Kramer et al. 2018). According to a systematic review of available studies and clinical trials on the effectiveness and safety of topical antimicrobial treatments for DFU, it is suggested that the use of an antimicrobial dressing instead of a non-antimicrobial dressing may contribute to DFU healing (Dumville et al. 2017). A new wave of antiseptics, such as polyhexamethylene biguanide and octenidine dihydrochloride, show better tolerability, being recommended for the treatment of chronic and infected DFU (Hubner, Siebert, and Kramer 2010; To et al. 2016).

NICE only recommends bio-engineered skin and negative pressure for DFU treatment (Table 1). Bio-engineered skin replaces the degraded extracellular matrix by a new one, promoting wound closure (Yazdanpanah, Nasiri, and Adarvish 2015). The only human- and human/animal-derived products approved by FDA are Apligraf and Dermagraft, and they both are contraindicated for infected wounds. They should be used as a complementary approach to standard care only when healing does not improve (NICE 2015).

NPWT is a non-invasive wound closure system that uses controlled and localized negative pressure to promote neovascularization, blood flow and extracellular matrix remodeling, necessary for wound healing (Greene et al. 2006; Ravanti and Kahari 2000; Gary Sibbald and Woo 2008). It has been used for decades and is one of the most commonly used complementary approaches applied to DFU patients (Sebastian Borys et al. 2019). NICE and international guidelines recommend NPWT for the treatment of DFU following surgical debridement (Apelqvist et al. 2017; Game et al. 2016; NICE 2015).

ES is believed to reproduce the natural electrical current that occurs in wounds, improving wound healing (Thakral et al. 2013) by stimulating the migration of different types of cells towards the wound exudate (Braddock, Campbell, and Zuder 1999), improving the blood flow at wound site; promoting the synthesis of collagen (Clark 1998; Singer and Clark 1999), and reducing inflammation (Odell and Sorgnard 2008; Sari et al. 2017; Sebastian et al. 2011). Despite these positive results, the use of ES is not recommended (Table 1) (NICE 2015), and more studies are required to fully understand the effects and mode of action of this therapy on wound healing.

Becaplermin is the only recombinant human platelet-derived growth factor approved for application to chronic diabetic wounds (LeGrand 1998; Wieman, Smiell, and Su 1998), contributing for the increase of diabetic patients with complete wound healing and lowering amputation risk (Martí-Carvajal et al. 2015). However, some studies associate its use with an increase in cancer development (Papanas and Maltezos 2010). Therefore, the potential risks of Becaplermin need to be carefully assessed by consistent clinical trials.

HBOT is used to increase oxygen delivery to ischemic tissues (Dunnill et al. 2017). However, recent clinical trials show that adjuvant HBOT has no significant advantage on wound healing when compared with standard care (Fedorko et al. 2016; Zhao et al. 2017; Santema et al. 2018). Therefore, its use is not recommended until the implementation of suitably clinical trials, aiming at establishing the role of this therapy in DFU treatment.

G-CSF is an endogenous hematopoietic growth factor that improves the function of both normal and defective neutrophils (Gough et al. 1997). Although some studies indicate a significant role of G-CSF in reducing lower extremity surgical interventions including amputation and the hospitalization period (Cruciani 2013; Xu and Liang 2016), given the high costs associated with its use and the lack of increased efficacy of G-CSF therapy described in most studies, its use as an complementary treatment is not recommended (Cruciani 2013; NICE 2015).

LLLT uses light to alter cellular function and molecular pathways, contributing for the reduction of ulcer size and for the improvement of wound healing (Li et al. 2018). Additional studies are needed to validate LLLT application to DFU treatment (Li et al. 2018; Tchanque-Fossuo et al. 2016). However, it shows the potential to become a portable and easy-to-use technique for the treatment of DFU with the advantage of being a minimally invasive technique (Li et al. 2018; Tchanque-Fossuo et al. 2016).

Bacteriophage therapy uses lytic bacteriophages to reduce or eliminate pathogenic bacteria (Mendes et al. 2014). DFI are recalcitrant to antibiotic therapy due to poor vascularization and the presence of resistant and biofilm-producing strains, which make them good targets for bacteriophage therapy (Mottola et al. 2016a, 2016b, 2016c). FDA has authorized the development of clinical trials using TP-102, a bacteriophage cocktail developed in Portugal (Mendes et al. 2014). Despite the numerous *in vitro* and *in vivo* studies and multiple clinical trials demonstrating that the use of bacteriophages can be useful and effective against DFI, regulatory and policy constraints hamper its clinical use (Furfaro, Payne, and Chang 2018). A European organization was created in 2009 to streamline a specific regulatory framework for phage therapy in Europe, and to support phage research and phage prophylactic and therapeutic applications (P.H.A.G.E. 2009).

In conclusion, there should be a focus on developing novel advanced therapies to promote DFU healing, to prevent its infection and treat DFI effectively. Studies and clinical trials should be designed to establish the role of advanced therapies in DFU treatment and proper therapeutic protocols (including guidelines for the identification of patients that would benefit from such treatments, the adequate dose to be applied, the ideal time-point to initiate treatment and its duration). In the long-term, these advanced therapeutics would contribute to decrease the costs associated with DM and to improve patient's quality of life.

REFERENCES

Abedon, S. T., S. J. Kuhl, B. G. Blasdel, and E. M. Kutter. 2011. "Phage treatment of human infections." *Bacteriophage* 1 (2): 66-85. https://doi.org/ 10. 4161/ bact.1.2.15845.

Abidia, A., G. Laden, G. Kuhan, B. F. Johnson, A. R. Wilkinson, P. M. Renwick, E. A. Masson, and P. T. McCollum. 2003. "The role of hyperbaric oxygen therapy in ischaemic diabetic lower extremity ulcers: a double-blind randomised-controlled trial." *Eur J Vasc Endovasc Surg* 25 (6): 513-8. https://doi.org/10.1053/ejvs.2002.1911.

Ackermann, H. W. 2009. "Phage classification and characterization." *Methods Mol Biol* 501: 127-40. https://doi.org/10.1007/978-1-60327-164-6_13.

Adunsky, A., A. Ohry, and Ddct Group. 2005. "Decubitus direct current treatment (DDCT) of pressure ulcers: results of a randomized double-blinded placebo controlled study." *Arch Gerontol Geriatr* 41 (3): 261-9. https://doi.org/10.1016/j.archger.2005.04.004.

Agrawal, K. S., A. V. Sarda, R. Shrotriya, M. Bachhav, V. Puri, and G. Nataraj. 2017. "Acetic acid dressings: Finding the Holy Grail for infected wound management." *Indian J Plast Surg* 50 (3): 273-280. https://doi.org/10.4103/ijps.IJPS_245_16.

Al Ghamdi, K. M., A. Kumar, and N. A. Moussa. 2012. "Low-level laser therapy: a useful technique for enhancing the proliferation of various cultured cells." *Lasers Med Sci* 27 (1): 237-49. https:// doi.org/ 10.1007/ s10103-011-0885-2.

Anders, N., and J. Wollensak. 1997. "Inadvertent use of chlorhexidine instead of balanced salt solution for intraocular irrigation." *J Cataract Refract Surg* 23 (6): 959-62.

Andrae, J., R. Gallini, and C. Betsholtz. 2008. "Role of platelet-derived growth factors in physiology and medicine." *Genes Dev* 22 (10): 1276-312. https:// doi.org/ 10.1101/ gad.1653708.

Apelqvist, J., C. Willy, A. M. Fagerdahl, M. Fraccalvieri, M. Malmsjo, A. Piaggesi, A. Probst, and P. Vowden. 2017. "EWMA Document: Negative Pressure Wound Therapy." *J Wound Care* 26 (Sup3): S1-S154. https:// doi.org/ 10.12968/ jowc.2017.26.Sup3.S1.

Armstrong, D. G., A. J. M. Boulton, and S. A. Bus. 2017. "Diabetic Foot Ulcers and Their Recurrence." *N Engl J Med* 376 (24): 2367-2375. https:// doi.org/10.1056/NEJMra1615439.

Armstrong, D. G., L. A. Lavery, and Consortium Diabetic Foot Study. 2005. "Negative pressure wound therapy after partial diabetic foot amputation: a multicentre, randomised controlled trial." *Lancet* 366 (9498): 1704-10. https://doi.org/10.1016/S0140-6736(05)67695-7.

Armstrong, D. G., L. A. Lavery, and L. B. Harkless. 1998. "Validation of a diabetic wound classification system. The contribution of depth, infection, and ischemia to risk of amputation." *Diabetes Care* 21 (5): 855-9. https://www.ncbi.nlm.nih.gov/pubmed/9589255.

Armstrong, D. G., L. A. Lavery, B. P. Nixon, and A. J. Boulton. 2004. "It's not what you put on, but what you take off: techniques for debriding and off-loading the diabetic foot wound." *Clin Infect Dis* 39 Suppl 2: S92-9. https://doi.org/10.1086/383269.

Asadi, M. R., G. Torkaman, M. Hedayati, M. R. Mohajeri-Tehrani, M. Ahmadi, and R. F. Gohardani. 2017. "Angiogenic effects of low-intensity cathodal direct current on ischemic diabetic foot ulcers: A randomized controlled trial." *Diabetes Res Clin Pract* 127: 147-155. https://doi.org/10.1016/j.diabres.2017.03.012.

Assimacopoulos, D. 1968. "Wound healing promotion by the use of negative electric current." *Am Surg* 34 (6): 423-31. https://www.ncbi.nlm.nih.gov/pubmed/5651495.

Avci, P., A. Gupta, M. Sadasivam, D. Vecchio, Z. Pam, N. Pam, and M. R. Hamblin. 2013. "Low-level laser (light) therapy (LLLT) in skin: stimulating, healing, restoring." *Semin Cutan Med Surg* 32 (1): 41-52. https://www.ncbi.nlm.nih.gov/pubmed/24049929.

Bakker, D. J. 2000. "Hyperbaric oxygen therapy and the diabetic foot." *Diabetes Metab Res Rev* 16 Suppl 1: S55-8. https://www.ncbi.nlm.nih.gov/pubmed/11054890.

Banwell, P. E., and L. Teot. 2003. "Topical negative pressure (TNP): the evolution of a novel wound therapy." *J Wound Care* 12 (1): 22-8. https://doi.org/10.12968/jowc.2003.12.1.26451.

Barolet, D. 2008. "Light-emitting diodes (LEDs) in dermatology." *Semin Cutan Med Surg* 27 (4): 227-38. https://doi.org/10.1016/j.sder.2008.08.003.

Barun, V. V., A. P. Ivanov, A. V. Volotovskaya, and V.S. Ulashchik. 2007. "Absorption spectra and light penetration depth of normal and pathologically altered human skin." *J Appl Spectrosc* 74(3): 430-39. https://doi.org/10.1007/s10812-007-0071-2.

Basford, J. R. 1995. "Low intensity laser therapy: still not an established clinical tool." *Lasers Surg Med* 16 (4): 331-42. https://www.ncbi.nlm.nih.gov/pubmed/7651054.

Beckmann, K. H., G. Meyer-Hamme, and S. Schroder. 2014. "Low level laser therapy for the treatment of diabetic foot ulcers: a critical survey." *Evid Based Complement Alternat Med* 2014: 626127. https://doi.org/10.1155/2014/626127.

Bennett, S. P., G. D. Griffiths, A. M. Schor, G. P. Leese, and S. L. Schor. 2003. "Growth factors in the treatment of diabetic foot ulcers." *Br J Surg* 90 (2): 133-46. https://doi.org/10.1002/bjs.4019.

Blakytny, R., and E. B. Jude. 2009. "Altered molecular mechanisms of diabetic foot ulcers." *Int J Low Extrem Wounds* 8 (2): 95-104. https://doi.org/10.1177/1534734609337151.

Bloom D. E., E. T. Cafiero, E. Jané-Llopis, S. Abrahams-Gessel, L. R. Bloom, S. Fathima, A. B. Feigl, T. Gaziano, M. Mowafi, A. Pandya, K. Prettner, L. Rosenberg, B. Seligman, A. Z. Stein, and C. Weinstein. 2011. *The global economic burden of noncommunicable diseases*

(Working Paper Series). Geneva: Harvard School of Public Health and World Economic Forum.

Blume, P. A., J. Walters, W. Payne, J. Ayala, and J. Lantis. 2008. "Comparison of negative pressure wound therapy using vacuum-assisted closure with advanced moist wound therapy in the treatment of diabetic foot ulcers: a multicenter randomized controlled trial." *Diabetes Care* 31 (4): 631-6. https://doi.org/10.2337/dc07-2196.

Bonner, J. C. 2004. "Regulation of PDGF and its receptors in fibrotic diseases." *Cytokine Growth Factor Rev* 15 (4): 255-73. https://doi.org/10.1016/j.cytogfr.2004.03.006.

Borgquist, O., R. Ingemansson, and M. Malmsjo. 2010. "Wound edge microvascular blood flow during negative-pressure wound therapy: examining the effects of pressures from -10 to -175 mmHg." *Plast Reconstr Surg* 125 (2): 502-9. https://doi.org/10.1097/PRS.0b013e3181c82e1f.

Borys, S., A. H. Ludwig-Slomczynska, M. Seweryn, J. Hohendorff, T. Koblik, J. Machlowska, B. Kiec-Wilk, P. Wolkow, and M. T. Malecki. 2019b. "Negative pressure wound therapy in the treatment of diabetic foot ulcers may be mediated through differential gene expression." *Acta Diabetol* 56 (1): 115-120. https://doi.org/10.1007/s00592-018-1223-y.

Borys, S., J. Hohendorff, C. Frankfurter, B. Kiec-Wilk, and M. T. Malecki. 2019a. "Negative pressure wound therapy use in diabetic foot syndrome - from mechanisms of action to clinical practice." *Eur J Clin Invest* 49 (4): e13067. https://doi.org/10.1111/eci.13067.

Boyanova, L., and I. Mitov. 2013. "Antibiotic resistance rates in causative agents of infections in diabetic patients: rising concerns." *Expert Rev Anti Infect Ther* 11 (4): 411-20. https://doi.org/10.1586/eri.13.19.

Braddock, M., C. J. Campbell, and D. Zuder. 1999. "Current therapies for wound healing: electrical stimulation, biological therapeutics, and the potential for gene therapy." *Int J Dermatol* 38 (11): 808-17. https://www.ncbi.nlm.nih.gov/pubmed/10583612.

Burrowes, B., D. R. Harper, J. Anderson, M. McConville, and M. C. Enright. 2011. "Bacteriophage therapy: potential uses in the control of antibiotic-resistant pathogens." *Expert Rev Anti Infect Ther* 9 (9): 775-85. https://doi.org/10.1586/eri.11.90.

Cavorsi, J., F. Vicari, D. J. Wirthlin, W. Ennis, R. Kirsner, S. M. O'Connell, J. Steinberg, and V. Falanga. 2006. "Best-practice algorithms for the use of a bilayered living cell therapy (Apligraf) in the treatment of lower-extremity ulcers." *Wound Repair Regen* 14 (2): 102-9. https://doi.org/10.1111/j.1743-6109.2006.00098.x.

Chen, C. E., J. Y. Ko, C. Y. Fong, and R. J. Juhn. 2010. "Treatment of diabetic foot infection with hyperbaric oxygen therapy." *Foot Ankle Surg* 16 (2): 91-5. https://doi.org/10.1016/j.fas.2009.06.002.

Chen, J., and R. P. Novick. 2009. "Phage-mediated intergeneric transfer of toxin genes." *Science* 323 (5910): 139-41. https://doi.org/10.1126/science.1164783.

Chen, S. J., C. T. Yu, Y. L. Cheng, S. Y. Yu, and H. C. Lo. 2007. "Effects of hyperbaric oxygen therapy on circulating interleukin-8, nitric oxide, and insulin-like growth factors in patients with type 2 diabetes mellitus." *Clin Biochem* 40 (1-2): 30-6. https://doi.org/10.1016/j.clinbiochem.2006.07.007.

Chin, Y. F., T. T. Huang, B. R. Hsu, L. C. Weng, and C. C. Wang. 2019. "Factors associated with foot ulcer self-management behaviours among hospitalised patients with diabetes." *J Clin Nurs* 28 (11-12): 2253-2264. https://doi.org/10.1111/jocn.14822.

Chuan, F., K. Tang, P. Jiang, B. Zhou, and X. He. 2015. "Reliability and validity of the perfusion, extent, depth, infection and sensation (PEDIS) classification system and score in patients with diabetic foot ulcer." *PLoS One* 10 (4): e0124739. https://doi.org/10.1371/journal.pone.0124739.

Chung, H., T. Dai, S. K. Sharma, Y. Y. Huang, J. D. Carroll, and M. R. Hamblin. 2012. "The nuts and bolts of low-level laser (light) therapy." *Ann Biomed Eng* 40 (2): 516-33. https://doi.org/10.1007/s10439-011-0454-7.

Clark, J. R., and J. B. March. 2006. "Bacteriophages and biotechnology: vaccines, gene therapy and antibacterials." *Trends Biotechnol* 24 (5): 212-8. https://doi.org/10.1016/j.tibtech.2006.03.003.

Clark, R. A. F. 1998. "Overview and General Considerations of Wound Repair." In *The Molecular and Cellular Biology of Wound Repair*, 3–33. Boston, MA: Springer US. https://doi.org/10.1007/978-1-4615-1795-5_1.

Cruciani, M., B. A. Lipsky, C. Mengoli, and F. de Lalla. 2013. "Granulocyte-colony stimulating factors as adjunctive therapy for diabetic foot infections." *Cochrane Database Syst Rev* (8): CD006810. https://doi.org/10.1002/14651858.CD006810.pub3.

Dabrowska, K., K. Switala-Jelen, A. Opolski, B. Weber-Dabrowska, and A. Gorski. 2005. "Bacteriophage penetration in vertebrates." *J Appl Microbiol* 98 (1): 7-13. https://doi.org/10.1111/j.1365-2672.2004.02422.x. https://www.ncbi.nlm.nih.gov/pubmed/15610412.

Dale, D. C., W. C. Liles, W. R. Summer, and S. Nelson. 1995. "Review: granulocyte colony-stimulating factor--role and relationships in infectious diseases." *J Infect Dis* 172 (4): 1061-75. https://www.ncbi.nlm.nih.gov/pubmed/7561181.

Davis, S. C., L. Martinez, and R. Kirsner. 2006. "The diabetic foot: the importance of biofilms and wound bed preparation." *Curr Diab Rep* 6 (6): 439-45. https://www.ncbi.nlm.nih.gov/pubmed/17118226.

de Lalla, F., R. Nicolin, and L. Lazzarini. 2000. "Safety and efficacy of recombinant granulocyte colony-stimulating factor as an adjunctive therapy for *Streptococcus pneumoniae* meningitis in non-neutropenic adult patients: a pilot study." *J Antimicrob Chemother* 46 (5): 843-6. https://www.ncbi.nlm.nih.gov/pubmed/11062212.

De, S. K., E. D. Reis, and M. D. Kerstein. 2002. "Wound treatment with human skin equivalent." *J Am Podiatr Med Assoc* 92 (1): 19-23. https://www.ncbi.nlm.nih.gov/pubmed/11796795.

del Pino-Sedeno, T., M. M. Trujillo-Martin, I. Andia, J. Aragon-Sanchez, E. Herrera-Ramos, F. J. Iruzubieta Barragan, and P. Serrano-Aguilar. 2019. "Platelet-rich plasma for the treatment of diabetic foot ulcers: A meta-analysis." *Wound Repair Regen* 27 (2): 170-182. https://doi.org/10.1111/wrr.12690.

Deuel, T. F., R. M. Senior, J. S. Huang, and G. L. Griffin. 1982. "Chemotaxis of monocytes and neutrophils to platelet-derived growth factor." *J Clin Invest* 69 (4): 1046-9. https://www.ncbi.nlm.nih.gov/pubmed/7076844.

Dolynchuk, K., P. Hull, L. Guenther, R. G. Sibbald, A. Brassard, M. Cooling, L. Delorme, W. Gulliver, D. H. Bourassa, V. Ho, B. Kunimoto, T. Overholt, K. Papp, and J. Tousignant. 1999. "The role of Apligraf in the treatment of venous leg ulcers." *Ostomy Wound Manage* 45 (1): 34-43. https://www.ncbi.nlm.nih.gov/pubmed/10085970.

Dowd, S. E., J. Delton Hanson, E. Rees, R. D. Wolcott, A. M. Zischau, Y. Sun, J. White, D. M. Smith, J. Kennedy, and C. E. Jones. 2011. "Survey of fungi and yeast in polymicrobial infections in chronic wounds." *J Wound Care* 20 (1): 40-7. https://doi.org/10.12968/jowc.2011.20.1.40.

Drulis-Kawa, Z., G. Majkowska-Skrobek, B. Maciejewska, A. S. Delattre, and R. Lavigne. 2012. "Learning from bacteriophages - advantages and limitations of phage and phage-encoded protein applications." *Curr Protein Pept Sci* 13 (8): 699-722. https://www.ncbi.nlm.nih.gov/pubmed/23305359.

Dumville, J. C., B. A. Lipsky, C. Hoey, M. Cruciani, M. Fiscon, and J. Xia. 2017. "Topical antimicrobial agents for treating foot ulcers in people with diabetes." *Cochrane Database Syst Rev* 6: CD011038. https://doi.org/10.1002/14651858.CD011038.pub2.

Dumville, J. C., R. J. Hinchliffe, N. Cullum, F. Game, N. Stubbs, M. Sweeting, and F. Peinemann. 2013. "Negative pressure wound therapy for treating foot wounds in people with diabetes mellitus." *Cochrane Database Syst Rev* (10): CD010318. https://doi.org/10.1002/14651858.CD010318.pub2.

Dunnill, C., T. Patton, J. Brennan, J. Barrett, M. Dryden, J. Cooke, D. Leaper, and N. T. Georgopoulos. 2017. "Reactive oxygen species (ROS) and wound healing: the functional role of ROS and emerging ROS-modulating technologies for augmentation of the healing process." *Int Wound J* 14 (1): 89-96. https://doi.org/10.1111/iwj.12557.

Duzgun, A. P., H. Z. Satir, O. Ozozan, B. Saylam, B. Kulah, and F. Coskun. 2008. "Effect of hyperbaric oxygen therapy on healing of diabetic foot ulcers." *J Foot Ankle Surg* 47 (6): 515-9. https://doi.org/10.1053/j.jfas.2008.08.002.

Edmonds, M., M. Bates, M. Doxford, A. Gough, and A. Foster. 2000. "New treatments in ulcer healing and wound infection." *Diabetes Metab Res Rev* 16 Suppl 1: S51-4. https://www.ncbi.nlm.nih.gov/pubmed/11054889.

Eleftheriadou, I., N. Tentolouris, V. Argiana, E. Jude, and A. J. Boulton. 2010. "Methicillin-resistant *Staphylococcus aureus* in diabetic foot infections." *Drugs* 70 (14): 1785-97. https://doi.org/10.2165/11538070-000000000-00000.

Eppley, B. L., J. E. Woodell, and J. Higgins. 2004. "Platelet quantification and growth factor analysis from platelet-rich plasma: implications for wound healing." *Plast Reconstr Surg* 114 (6): 1502-8. https://www.ncbi.nlm.nih.gov/pubmed/15509939.

Everett, E., and N. Mathioudakis. 2018. "Update on management of diabetic foot ulcers." *Ann N Y Acad Sci* 1411 (1): 153-165. https://doi.org/10.1111/nyas.13569.

Faglia, E., F. Favales, A. Aldeghi, P. Calia, A. Quaratiello, G. Oriani, M. Michael, P. Campagnoli, and A. Morabito. 1996. "Adjunctive systemic hyperbaric oxygen therapy in treatment of severe prevalently ischemic diabetic foot ulcer. A randomized study." *Diabetes Care* 19 (12): 1338-43. https://www.ncbi.nlm.nih.gov/pubmed/8941460.

Fair, R. J., and Y. Tor. 2014. "Antibiotics and bacterial resistance in the 21st century." *Perspect Medicin Chem* 6: 25-64. https://doi.org/10.4137/PMC.S14459.

Falanga, V. 2005. "Wound healing and its impairment in the diabetic foot." *Lancet* 366 (9498): 1736-43. https://doi.org/10.1016/S0140-6736(05)67700-8.

Fedorko, L., J. M. Bowen, W. Jones, G. Oreopoulos, R. Goeree, R. B. Hopkins, and D. J. O'Reilly. 2016. "Hyperbaric Oxygen Therapy does not reduce indications for amputation in patients with Diabetes with nonhealing ulcers of the lower limb: a prospective, double-blind, randomized controlled clinical trial." *Diabetes Care* 39 (3): 392-9. https://doi.org/10.2337/dc15-2001.

Feedar, J. A., L. C. Kloth, and G. D. Gentzkow. 1991. "Chronic dermal ulcer healing enhanced with monophasic pulsed electrical stimulation." *Phys Ther* 71 (9): 639-49. https://www.ncbi.nlm.nih.gov/pubmed/1881954.

Feiner, R., T. Argov, L. Rabinovich, N. Sigal, I. Borovok, and A. A. Herskovits. 2015. "A new perspective on lysogeny: prophages as active regulatory switches of bacteria." *Nat Rev Microbiol* 13 (10): 641-50. https://doi.org/10.1038/nrmicro3527.

Fernando, M. E., R. M. Seneviratne, Y. M. Tan, P. A. Lazzarini, K. S. Sangla, M. Cunningham, P. G. Buttner, and J. Golledge. 2016. "Intensive *versus* conventional glycaemic control for treating diabetic foot ulcers." *Cochrane Database Syst Rev* (1): CD010764. https://doi.org/10.1002/14651858.CD010764.pub2.

Fish, R., E. Kutter, G. Wheat, B. Blasdel, M. Kutateladze, and S. Kuhl. 2018. "Compassionate use of bacteriophage therapy for foot ulcer treatment as an effective step for moving toward clinical trials." *Methods Mol Biol* 1693: 159-170. https://doi.org/10.1007/978-1-4939-7395-8_14.

Foster, T. E., B. L. Puskas, B. R. Mandelbaum, M. B. Gerhardt, and S. A. Rodeo. 2009. "Platelet-rich plasma: from basic science to clinical applications." *Am J Sports Med* 37 (11): 2259-72. https://doi.org/10.1177/0363546509349921.

Foulds, I. S., and A. T. Barker. 1983. "Human skin battery potentials and their possible role in wound healing." *Br J Dermatol* 109 (5): 515-22. https://www.ncbi.nlm.nih.gov/pubmed/6639877.

Frechette, J. P., I. Martineau, and G. Gagnon. 2005. "Platelet-rich plasmas: growth factor content and roles in wound healing." *J Dent Res* 84 (5): 434-9. https://doi.org/10.1177/154405910508400507.

Furfaro, L. L., M. S. Payne, and B. J. Chang. 2018. "Bacteriophage therapy: clinical trials and regulatory hurdles." *Front Cell Infect Microbiol* 8: 376. https://doi.org/10.3389/fcimb.2018.00376.

Game, F. L., C. Attinger, A. Hartemann, R. J. Hinchliffe, M. Londahl, P. E. Price, W. J. Jeffcoate, and Foot International Working Group on the Diabetic. 2016a. "IWGDF guidance on use of interventions to enhance the healing of chronic ulcers of the foot in diabetes." *Diabetes Metab Res Rev* 32 Suppl 1: 75-83. https://doi.org/10.1002/dmrr.2700.

Game, F. L., J. Apelqvist, C. Attinger, A. Hartemann, R. J. Hinchliffe, M. Londahl, P. E. Price, W. J. Jeffcoate, and Foot International Working Group on the Diabetic. 2016b. "Effectiveness of interventions to enhance healing of chronic ulcers of the foot in diabetes: a systematic review." *Diabetes Metab Res Rev* 32 Suppl 1: 154-68. https://doi.org/10.1002/dmrr.2707.

Garfein E. 2009. "Skin replacement products and markets" In *Biomaterials for Treating Skin Loss*, D.P. Orgill and C. Blanco, 256 p. Cambridge: Woodhead Publishing.

Gary Sibbald, R., and K. Y. Woo. 2008. "The biology of chronic foot ulcers in persons with diabetes." *Diabetes Metab Res Rev* 24 Suppl 1: S25-30. https://doi.org/10.1002/dmrr.847.

Geerlings, S. E., and A. I. Hoepelman. 1999. "Immune dysfunction in patients with Diabetes *mellitus* (DM)." *FEMS Immunol Med Microbiol* 26 (3-4): 259-65. https://doi.org/10.1111/j.1574-695X.1999.tb01397.x.

Golebiewska, E. M., and A. W. Poole. 2015. "Platelet secretion: from haemostasis to wound healing and beyond." *Blood Rev* 29 (3): 153-62. https://doi.org/10.1016/j.blre.2014.10.003.

Gottrup, F. 2005. "Management of the diabetic foot: surgical and organisational aspects." *Horm Metab Res* 37 Suppl 1: 69-75. https://doi.org/10.1055/s-2005-861377.

Gough, A., M. Clapperton, N. Rolando, A. V. Foster, J. Philpott-Howard, and M. E. Edmonds. 1997. "Randomised placebo-controlled trial of granulocyte-colony stimulating factor in diabetic foot infection." *Lancet* 350 (9081): 855-9. https://doi.org/10.1016/S0140-6736(97)04495-4.

Grazul-Bilska, A. T., M. L. Johnson, J. J. Bilski, D. A. Redmer, L. P. Reynolds, A. Abdullah, and K. M. Abdullah. 2003. "Wound healing: the role of growth factors." *Drugs Today (Barc)* 39 (10): 787-800. https://www.ncbi.nlm.nih.gov/pubmed/14668934.

Greaves, N. S., K. J. Ashcroft, M. Baguneid, and A. Bayat. 2013. "Current understanding of molecular and cellular mechanisms in fibroplasia and angiogenesis during acute wound healing." *J Dermatol Sci* 72 (3): 206-17. https://doi.org/10.1016/j.jdermsci.2013.07.008.

Greene, A. K., M. Puder, R. Roy, D. Arsenault, S. Kwei, M. A. Moses, and D. P. Orgill. 2006. "Microdeformational wound therapy: effects on angiogenesis and matrix metalloproteinases in chronic wounds of 3 debilitated patients." *Ann Plast Surg* 56 (4): 418-22. https://doi.org/10.1097/01.sap.0000202831.43294.02.

Han, G., and R. Ceilley. 2017. "Chronic wound healing: a review of current management and treatments." *Adv Ther* 34 (3): 599-610. https://doi.org/10.1007/s12325-017-0478-y.

Hanft, J. R., and M. S. Surprenant. 2002. "Healing of chronic foot ulcers in diabetic patients treated with a human fibroblast-derived dermis." *J Foot Ankle Surg* 41 (5): 291-9. https://www.ncbi.nlm.nih.gov/pubmed/12400712.

Haq, I. U., W. N. Chaudhry, M. N. Akhtar, S. Andleeb, and I. Qadri. 2012. "Bacteriophages and their implications on future biotechnology: a review." *Virol J* 9: 9. https://doi.org/10.1186/1743-422X-9-9.

Hartung, T. 1999. "Granulocyte colony-stimulating factor: its potential role in infectious disease." *AIDS* 13 Suppl 2: S3-9. https://www.ncbi.nlm.nih.gov/pubmed/10596675.

Hasan, M. Y., R. Teo, and A. Nather. 2015. "Negative-pressure wound therapy for management of diabetic foot wounds: a review of the mechanism of action, clinical applications, and recent developments." *Diabet Foot Ankle* 6: 27618. https://doi.org/10.3402/dfa.v6.27618.

He, C., S. C. Medley, T. Hu, M. E. Hinsdale, F. Lupu, R. Virmani, and L. E. Olson. 2015. "PDGFRbeta signalling regulates local inflammation and synergizes with hypercholesterolaemia to promote atherosclerosis." *Nat Commun* 6: 7770. https://doi.org/10.1038/ncomms8770.

Heldin, C. H., J. Lennartsson, and B. Westermark. 2018. "Involvement of platelet-derived growth factor ligands and receptors in tumorigenesis." *J Intern Med* 283 (1): 16-44. https://doi.org/10.1111/joim.12690.

Hermann, T. 2007. "Aminoglycoside antibiotics: old drugs and new therapeutic approaches." *Cell Mol Life Sci* 64 (14): 1841-52. https://doi.org/10.1007/s00018-007-7034-x.

Heyneman, C. A., and C. Lawless-Liday. 2002. "Using hyperbaric oxygen to treat diabetic foot ulcers: safety and effectiveness." *Crit Care Nurse* 22 (6): 52-60. https://www.ncbi.nlm.nih.gov/pubmed/12518568.

Hirsch, T., H. M. Seipp, F. Jacobsen, O. Goertz, H. U. Steinau, and L. Steinstraesser. 2010. "Antiseptics in surgery." *Eplasty* 10: e39. https://www.ncbi.nlm.nih.gov/pubmed/20526354.

Hobizal, K. B., and D. K. Wukich. 2012. "Diabetic foot infections: current concept review." *Diabet Foot Ankle* 3. https://doi.org/10.3402/dfa.v3i0.18409.

Hollinger, J. O., C. E. Hart, S. N. Hirsch, S. Lynch, and G. E. Friedlaender. 2008. "Recombinant human platelet-derived growth factor: biology and clinical applications." *J Bone Joint Surg Am* 90 Suppl 1: 48-54. https://doi.org/10.2106/JBJS.G.01231.

Houghton, P. E. 2017. "Electrical stimulation therapy to promote healing of chronic wounds: a review of reviews." *Chronic Wound Care Manag Res* 4: 25–44. https://doi.org/10.2147/CWCMR.S101323.

Houghton, P. E., K. E. Campbell, C. H. Fraser, C. Harris, D. H. Keast, P. J. Potter, K. C. Hayes, and M. G. Woodbury. 2010. "Electrical stimulation therapy increases rate of healing of pressure ulcers in community-dwelling people with spinal cord injury." *Arch Phys Med Rehabil* 91 (5): 669-78. https://doi.org/10.1016/j.apmr.2009.12.026.

Houreld, N., and H. Abrahamse. 2010. "Low-intensity laser irradiation stimulates wound healing in diabetic wounded fibroblast cells (WS1)." *Diabetes Technol Ther* 12 (12): 971-8. https://doi.org/10.1089/dia.2010.0039.

Huang, C., T. Leavitt, L. R. Bayer, and D. P. Orgill. 2014. "Effect of negative pressure wound therapy on wound healing." *Curr Probl Surg* 51 (7): 301-31. https://doi.org/10.1067/j.cpsurg.2014.04.001.

Hubner, N. O., J. Siebert, and A. Kramer. 2010. "Octenidine dihydrochloride, a modern antiseptic for skin, mucous membranes and wounds." *Skin Pharmacol Physiol* 23 (5): 244-58. https://doi.org/10.1159/000314699.

Huys, I., J. P. Pirnay, R. Lavigne, S. Jennes, D. De Vos, M. Casteels, and G. Verbeken. 2013. "Paving a regulatory pathway for phage therapy. Europe should muster the resources to financially, technically and legally support the introduction of phage therapy." *EMBO Rep* 14 (11): 951-4. https://doi.org/10.1038/embor.2013.163.

Ince, P., F. L. Game, and W. J. Jeffcoate. 2007. "Rate of healing of neuropathic ulcers of the foot in diabetes and its relationship to ulcer duration and ulcer area." *Diabetes Care* 30 (3): 660-3. https://doi.org/10.2337/dc06-2043.

Ince, P., Z. G. Abbas, J. K. Lutale, A. Basit, S. M. Ali, F. Chohan, S. Morbach, J. Mollenberg, F. L. Game, and W. J. Jeffcoate. 2008. "Use of the SINBAD classification system and score in comparing outcome of foot ulcer management on three continents." *Diabetes Care* 31 (5): 964-7. https://doi.org/10.2337/dc07-2367.

Jaffe, L. F., and J. W. Vanable, Jr. 1984. "Electric fields and wound healing." *Clin Dermatol* 2 (3): 34-44. https://www.ncbi.nlm.nih.gov/pubmed/6336255.

Junka, A., M. Bartoszewicz, D. Smutnicka, A. Secewicz, and P. Szymczyk. 2014. "Efficacy of antiseptics containing povidone-iodine, octenidine dihydrochloride and ethacridine lactate against biofilm formed by *Pseudomonas aeruginosa* and *Staphylococcus aureus* measured with the novel biofilm-oriented antiseptics test." *Int Wound J* 11 (6): 730-4. https://doi.org/10.1111/iwj.12057.

Kajagar, B. M., A. S. Godhi, A. Pandit, and S. Khatri. 2012. "Efficacy of low level laser therapy on wound healing in patients with chronic diabetic foot ulcers-a randomised control trial." *Indian J Surg* 74 (5): 359-63. https://doi.org/10.1007/s12262-011-0393-4.

Karu, T. 1989. "Photobiology of low-power laser effects." *Health Phys* 56 (5): 691-704. https://www.ncbi.nlm.nih.gov/pubmed/2651364.

Karu, T. I., and S. F. Kolyakov. 2005. "Exact action spectra for cellular responses relevant to phototherapy." *Photomed Laser Surg* 23 (4): 355-61. https://doi.org/10.1089/pho.2005.23.355.

Karu, T. I., L. V. Pyatibrat, and G. S. Kalendo. 2004. "Photobiological modulation of cell attachment via cytochrome c oxidase." *Photochem Photobiol Sci* 3 (2): 211-6. https://doi.org/10.1039/b306126d.

Kaviani, A., G. E. Djavid, L. Ataie-Fashtami, M. Fateh, M. Ghodsi, M. Salami, N. Zand, N. Kashef, and B. Larijani. 2011. "A randomized clinical trial on the effect of low-level laser therapy on chronic diabetic foot wound healing: a preliminary report." *Photomed Laser Surg* 29 (2): 109-14. https://doi.org/10.1089/pho.2009.2680.

Kavitha, K. V., S. Tiwari, V. B. Purandare, S. Khedkar, S. S. Bhosale, and A. G. Unnikrishnan. 2014. "Choice of wound care in diabetic foot ulcer: A practical approach." *World J Diabetes* 5 (4): 546-56. https://doi.org/10.4239/wjd.v5.i4.546.

Kazemi-Khoo, N. 2006. "Successful treatment of diabetic foot ulcers with low-level laser therapy." *The Foot.* 16(4): 184-187. http://dx.doi.org/10.1016/j.foot.2006.05.004.

Kessler, L., P. Bilbault, F. Ortega, C. Grasso, R. Passemard, D. Stephan, M. Pinget, and F. Schneider. 2003. "Hyperbaric oxygenation accelerates the healing rate of nonischemic chronic diabetic foot ulcers: a prospective randomized study." *Diabetes Care* 26 (8): 2378-82. https://www.ncbi.nlm.nih.gov/pubmed/12882865.

Khashim, Z., S. Samuel, N. Duraisamy, and K. Krishnan. 2019. "Potential biomolecules and current treatment technologies for diabetic foot ulcer: an overview." *Curr Diabetes Rev* 15 (1): 2-14. https://doi.org/10.2174/1573399813666170519102406.

Knezevic, P., and O. Petrovic. 2008. "A colorimetric microtiter plate method for assessment of phage effect on *Pseudomonas aeruginosa* biofilm." *J Microbiol Methods* 74 (2-3): 114-8. https://doi.org/10.1016/j.mimet.2008.03.005.

Kramer, A., J. Dissemond, S. Kim, C. Willy, D. Mayer, R. Papke, F. Tuchmann, and O. Assadian. 2018. "Consensus on Wound Antisepsis: Update 2018." *Skin Pharmacol Physiol* 31 (1): 28-58. https://doi.org/10.1159/000481545.

Krautheim, A. B., T. H. Jermann, and A. J. Bircher. 2004. "Chlorhexidine anaphylaxis: case report and review of the literature." *Contact*

Dermatitis 50 (3): 113-6. https://doi.org/10.1111/j.0105-1873.2004.00308.x.

Labrie, S. J., J. E. Samson, and S. Moineau. 2010. "Bacteriophage resistance mechanisms." *Nat Rev Microbiol* 8 (5): 317-27. https://doi.org/10.1038/nrmicro2315.

Landau, Z., M. Migdal, A. Lipovsky, and R. Lubart. 2011. "Visible light-induced healing of diabetic or venous foot ulcers: a placebo-controlled double-blind study." *Photomed Laser Surg* 29 (6): 399-404. https://doi.org/10.1089/pho.2010.2858.

Langer, A., and W. Rogowski. 2009. "Systematic review of economic evaluations of human cell-derived wound care products for the treatment of venous leg and diabetic foot ulcers." *BMC Health Serv Res* 9: 115. https://doi.org/10.1186/1472-6963-9-115.

LeGrand, E. K. 1998. "Preclinical promise of becaplermin (rhPDGF-BB) in wound healing." *Am J Surg* 176 (2A Suppl): 48S-54S. https://www.ncbi.nlm.nih.gov/pubmed/9777972.

Li, L., G. Takemura, Y. Li, S. Miyata, M. Esaki, H. Okada, H. Kanamori, A. Ogino, R. Maruyama, M. Nakagawa, S. Minatoguchi, T. Fujiwara, and H. Fujiwara. 2007. "Granulocyte colony-stimulating factor improves left ventricular function of doxorubicin-induced cardiomyopathy." *Lab Invest* 87 (5): 440-55. https://doi.org/10.1038/labinvest.3700530.

Li, S., C. Wang, B. Wang, L. Liu, L. Tang, D. Liu, G. Yang, and L. Zhang. 2018. "Efficacy of low-level light therapy for treatment of diabetic foot ulcer: A systematic review and meta-analysis of randomized controlled trials." *Diabetes Res Clin Pract* 143: 215-224. https://doi.org/10.1016/j.diabres.2018.07.014.

Lipovsky, A., Y. Nitzan, A. Gedanken, and R. Lubart. 2010. "Visible light-induced killing of bacteria as a function of wavelength: implication for wound healing." *Lasers Surg Med* 42 (6): 467-72. https://doi.org/10.1002/lsm.20948.

Lipsky, B. A., A. R. Berendt, H. G. Deery, J. M. Embil, W. S. Joseph, A. W. Karchmer, J. L. LeFrock, D. P. Lew, J. T. Mader, C. Norden, J. S. Tan, and America Infectious Diseases Society of. 2004. "Diagnosis and treatment of diabetic foot infections." *Clin Infect Dis* 39 (7): 885-910. https://doi.org/10.1086/424846.

Lipsky, B. A., A. R. Berendt, P. B. Cornia, J. C. Pile, E. J. Peters, D. G. Armstrong, H. G. Deery, J. M. Embil, W. S. Joseph, A. W. Karchmer, M. S. Pinzur, E. Senneville, and America Infectious Diseases Society of. 2012. "2012 Infectious Diseases Society of America clinical practice guideline for the diagnosis and treatment of diabetic foot infections." *Clin Infect Dis* 54 (12): e132-73. https://doi.org/10.1093/cid/cis346.

Lipsky, B. A., and A. R. Berendt. 2010. "Hyperbaric oxygen therapy for diabetic foot wounds: has hope hurdled hype?" *Diabetes Care* 33 (5): 1143-5. https://doi.org/10.2337/dc10-0393.

Lipsky, B. A., J. Aragon-Sanchez, M. Diggle, J. Embil, S. Kono, L. Lavery, E. Senneville, V. Urbancic-Rovan, S. Van Asten, Foot International Working Group on the Diabetic, and E. J. Peters. 2016. "IWGDF guidance on the diagnosis and management of foot infections in persons with diabetes." *Diabetes Metab Res Rev* 32 Suppl 1: 45-74. https://doi.org/10.1002/dmrr.2699.

Litscher, G. 2012. "Integrative laser medicine and high-tech acupuncture at the medical university of graz, austria, europe." *Evid Based Complement Alternat Med* 2012: 103109. https://doi.org/10.1155/2012/103109.

Liu, H., R. Colavitti, Rovira, II, and T. Finkel. 2005. "Redox-dependent transcriptional regulation." *Circ Res* 97 (10): 967-74. https://doi.org/10.1161/01.RES.0000188210.72062.10.

Liu, Z., J. C. Dumville, R. J. Hinchliffe, N. Cullum, F. Game, N. Stubbs, M. Sweeting, and F. Peinemann. 2018. "Negative pressure wound therapy for treating foot wounds in people with Diabetes *mellitus*." *Cochrane Database Syst Rev* 10: CD010318. https://doi.org/10.1002/14651858.CD010318.pub3.

Lopes, L., O. Setia, A. Aurshina, S. Liu, H. Hu, T. Isaji, H. Liu, T. Wang, S. Ono, X. Guo, B. Yatsula, J. Guo, Y. Gu, T. Navarro, and A. Dardik. 2018. "Stem cell therapy for diabetic foot ulcers: a review of preclinical and clinical research." *Stem Cell Res Ther* 9 (1): 188. https://doi.org/10.1186/s13287-018-0938-6.

Lu, T. K., and J. J. Collins. 2007. "Dispersing biofilms with engineered enzymatic bacteriophage." *Proc Natl Acad Sci U S A* 104 (27): 11197-202. https://doi.org/10.1073/pnas.0704624104.

Lundeberg, T. C., S. V. Eriksson, and M. Malm. 1992. "Electrical nerve stimulation improves healing of diabetic ulcers." *Ann Plast Surg* 29 (4): 328-31. https://www.ncbi.nlm.nih.gov/pubmed/1466529.

Machado, A. F., R. E. Liebano, F. Furtado, B. Hochman, and L. M. Ferreira. 2016. "Effect of high- and low-frequency transcutaneous electrical nerve stimulation on angiogenesis and myofibroblast proliferation in acute excisional wounds in rat skin." *Adv Skin Wound Care* 29 (8): 357-63. https://doi.org/10.1097/01.ASW.0000488721. 83423.f3.

Makarova, K. S., D. H. Haft, R. Barrangou, S. J. Brouns, E. Charpentier, P. Horvath, S. Moineau, F. J. Mojica, Y. I. Wolf, A. F. Yakunin, J. van der Oost, and E. V. Koonin. 2011. "Evolution and classification of the CRISPR-Cas systems." *Nat Rev Microbiol* 9 (6): 467-77. https://doi.org/10.1038/nrmicro2577.

Mansbridge, J. 1998. "Skin substitutes to enhance wound healing." *Expert Opin Investig Drugs* 7 (5): 803-9. https://doi.org/10.1517/13543784.7.5.803.

Mansbridge, J., K. Liu, R. Patch, K. Symons, and E. Pinney. 1998. "Three-dimensional fibroblast culture implant for the treatment of diabetic foot ulcers: metabolic activity and therapeutic range." *Tissue Eng* 4 (4): 403-14. https://doi.org/10.1089/ten.1998.4.403.

Margolis, D. J., C. Bartus, O. Hoffstad, S. Malay, and J. A. Berlin. 2005. "Effectiveness of recombinant human platelet-derived growth factor for the treatment of diabetic neuropathic foot ulcers." *Wound Repair Regen* 13(6):531-6. https://doi.org/10.1111/j.1524-475X.2005.00074.x.

Marston, W. A. 2004. "Dermagraft, a bioengineered human dermal equivalent for the treatment of chronic nonhealing diabetic foot ulcer." *Expert Rev Med Devices* 1 (1): 21-31. https://doi.org/10.1586/17434440.1.1.21.

Marston, W. A., and Group Dermagraft Diabetic Foot Ulcer Study. 2006. "Risk factors associated with healing chronic diabetic foot ulcers: the importance of hyperglycemia." *Ostomy Wound Manage* 52 (3): 26-8, 30, 32 passim. https://www.ncbi.nlm.nih.gov/pubmed/16567857.

Marston, W. A., J. Hanft, P. Norwood, R. Pollak, and Group Dermagraft Diabetic Foot Ulcer Study. 2003. "The efficacy and safety of Dermagraft in improving the healing of chronic diabetic foot ulcers: results of a prospective randomized trial." *Diabetes Care* 26 (6): 1701-5. https://www.ncbi.nlm.nih.gov/pubmed/12766097.

Martí-Carvajal, A. J., C. Gluud, S. Nicola, D. Simancas-Racines, L. Reveiz, P. Oliva, and J. Cedeno-Taborda. 2015. "Growth factors for treating diabetic foot ulcers." *Cochrane Database Syst Rev* (10): CD008548. https://doi.org/10.1002/14651858.CD008548.pub2.

Mat Saad, A. Z., T. L. Khoo, and A. S. Halim. 2013. "Wound bed preparation for chronic diabetic foot ulcers." *ISRN Endocrinol* 2013: 608313. https://doi.org/10.1155/2013/608313.

McDonnell, G., and A. D. Russell. 1999. "Antiseptics and disinfectants: activity, action, and resistance." *Clin Microbiol Rev* 12 (1): 147-79. https://www.ncbi.nlm.nih.gov/pubmed/9880479.

Mendes, J. J., A. Marques-Costa, C. Vilela, J. Neves, N. Candeias, P. Cavaco-Silva, and J. Melo-Cristino. 2012. "Clinical and bacteriological survey of diabetic foot infections in Lisbon." *Diabetes Res Clin Pract* 95 (1): 153-61. https://doi.org/10.1016/j.diabres.2011.10.001.

Mendes, J. J., C. Leandro, C. Mottola, R. Barbosa, F. A. Silva, M. Oliveira, C. L. Vilela, J. Melo-Cristino, A. Gorski, M. Pimentel, C. Sao-Jose, P. Cavaco-Silva, and M. Garcia. 2014. "*In vitro* design of a novel lytic bacteriophage cocktail with therapeutic potential against organisms causing diabetic foot infections." *J Med Microbiol* 63 (Pt 8): 1055-65. https://doi.org/10.1099/jmm.0.071753-0.

Menke, N. B., K. R. Ward, T. M. Witten, D. G. Bonchev, and R. F. Diegelmann. 2007. "Impaired wound healing." *Clin Dermatol* 25 (1): 19-25. https://doi.org/10.1016/j.clindermatol.2006.12.005.

Milstone, A. M., C. L. Passaretti, and T. M. Perl. 2008. "Chlorhexidine: expanding the armamentarium for infection control and prevention." *Clin Infect Dis* 46 (2): 274-81. https://doi.org/10.1086/524736.

Minatel, D. G., M. A. Frade, S. C. Franca, and C. S. Enwemeka. 2009. "Phototherapy promotes healing of chronic diabetic leg ulcers that failed to respond to other therapies." *Lasers Surg Med* 41 (6): 433-41. https://doi.org/10.1002/lsm.20789.

Minatoguchi, S., G. Takemura, X. H. Chen, N. Wang, Y. Uno, M. Koda, M. Arai, Y. Misao, C. Lu, K. Suzuki, K. Goto, A. Komada, T. Takahashi, K. Kosai, T. Fujiwara, and H. Fujiwara. 2004. "Acceleration of the healing process and myocardial regeneration may be important as a mechanism of improvement of cardiac function and remodeling by postinfarction granulocyte colony-stimulating factor treatment." *Circulation* 109 (21): 2572-80. https://doi.org/10.1161/01.CIR.0000129770.93985.3E.

Morozova, V. V., V. V. Vlassov, and N. V. Tikunova. 2018. "Applications of bacteriophages in the treatment of localized infections in humans." *Front Microbiol* 9: 1696. https://doi.org/10.3389/fmicb.2018.01696.

Mottola, C., C. S. Matias, J. J. Mendes, J. Melo-Cristino, L. Tavares, P. Cavaco-Silva, and M. Oliveira. 2016a. "Susceptibility patterns of *Staphylococcus aureus* biofilms in diabetic foot infections." *BMC Microbiol* 16 (1): 119. https://doi.org/10.1186/s12866-016-0737-0.

Mottola, C., J. J. Mendes, J. M. Cristino, P. Cavaco-Silva, L. Tavares, and M. Oliveira. 2016b. "Polymicrobial biofilms by diabetic foot clinical isolates." *Folia Microbiol (Praha)* 61 (1): 35-43. https://doi.org/10.1007/s12223-015-0401-3.

Mottola, C., T. Semedo-Lemsaddek, J. J. Mendes, J. Melo-Cristino, L. Tavares, P. Cavaco-Silva, and M. Oliveira. 2016c. "Molecular typing, virulence traits and antimicrobial resistance of diabetic foot staphylococci." *J Biomed Sci* 23: 33. https://doi.org/10.1186/s12929-016-0250-7.

Mulder, G., M. Tenenhaus, and G. F. D'Souza. 2014. "Reduction of diabetic foot ulcer healing times through use of advanced treatment modalities." *Int J Low Extrem Wounds* 13 (4): 335-46. https://doi.org/10.1177/1534734614557925.

Murata, A. 2003. "Granulocyte colony-stimulating factor as the expecting sword for the treatment of severe sepsis." *Curr Pharm Des* 9 (14): 1115-20. https://www.ncbi.nlm.nih.gov/pubmed/12769751.

Murdoch, R., K. M. Lagan. 2013. "The role of povidone and cadexomer iodine in the management of acute and chronic wounds." *Phys Ther Rev* 18(3): 207-216. https://doi.org/10.1179/1743288X13Y.0000000082.

Nagai, M. K., and J. M. Embil. 2002. "Becaplermin: recombinant platelet derived growth factor, a new treatment for healing diabetic foot ulcers." *Expert Opin Biol Ther* 2 (2): 211-8. https://doi.org/10.1517/14712598.2.2.211.

Nain, P. S., S. K. Uppal, R. Garg, K. Bajaj, and S. Garg. 2011. "Role of negative pressure wound therapy in healing of diabetic foot ulcers." *J Surg Tech Case Rep* 3 (1): 17-22. https://doi.org/10.4103/2006-8808.78466.

Nelson, S., A. M. Heyder, J. Stone, M. G. Bergeron, S. Daugherty, G. Peterson, N. Fotheringham, W. Welch, S. Milwee, and R. Root. 2000. "A randomized controlled trial of filgrastim for the treatment of hospitalized patients with multilobar pneumonia." *J Infect Dis* 182 (3): 970-3. https://doi.org/10.1086/315775.

Newton, D. J., F. Khan, J. J. Belch, M. R. Mitchell, and G. P. Leese. 2002. "Blood flow changes in diabetic foot ulcers treated with dermal replacement therapy." *J Foot Ankle Surg* 41 (4): 233-7. https://www.ncbi.nlm.nih.gov/pubmed/12194513.

NICE. 2015. "Diabetic foot problems: prevention and management" National Institute for Health and Care Excellence: Clinical Guidelines. London. https://www.nice.org.uk/guidance/ng19.

Noor, S., M. Zubair, and J. Ahmad. 2015. "Diabetic foot ulcer - a review on pathophysiology, classification and microbial etiology." *Diabetes Metab Syndr* 9 (3): 192-9. https://doi.org/10.1016/j.dsx.2015.04.007.

Nuccitelli, R., P. Nuccitelli, S. Ramlatchan, R. Sanger, and P. J. Smith. 2008. "Imaging the electric field associated with mouse and human skin wounds." *Wound Repair Regen* 16 (3): 432-41. https://doi.org/10.1111/j.1524-475X.2008.00389.x.

Odell, R. H., Jr., and R. E. Sorgnard. 2008. "Anti-inflammatory effects of electronic signal treatment." *Pain Physician* 11 (6): 891-907. https://www.ncbi.nlm.nih.gov/pubmed/19057635.

Osmundsen, P. E. 1982. "Contact dermatitis to chlorhexidine." *Contact Dermatitis* 8 (2): 81-3. https://www.ncbi.nlm.nih.gov/pubmed/6461508.

P.H.A.G.E. *Phages for Human Applications Group Europe.* 2009. Accessed May 29, 2019. http://www.p-h-a-g-e.org.

Panayi, A. C., T. Leavitt, and D. P. Orgill. 2017. "Evidence Based Review of Negative Pressure Wound Therapy." *World J Dermatol* 6 (1): 1-16. https://doi.org/10.5314/wjd.v6.i1.1.

Papanas, N., and E. Maltezos. 2010. "Benefit-risk assessment of becaplermin in the treatment of diabetic foot ulcers." *Drug Saf* 33 (6): 455-61. https://doi.org/10.2165/11534570-000000000-00000.

Parracho, H. M., B. H. Burrowes, M. C. Enright, M. L. McConville, and D. R. Harper. 2012. "The role of regulated clinical trials in the development of bacteriophage therapeutics." *J Mol Genet Med* 6: 279-86. https://www.ncbi.nlm.nih.gov/pubmed/22872803.

Peck, K. R., D. W. Son, J. H. Song, S. Kim, M. D. Oh, and K. W. Choe. 2001. "Enhanced neutrophil functions by recombinant human granulocyte colony-stimulating factor in diabetic patients with foot infections *in vitro*." *J Korean Med Sci* 16 (1): 39-44. https://doi.org/10.3346/jkms.2001.16.1.39.

Peplow, P. V., T. Y. Chung, B. Ryan, and G. D. Baxter. 2011. "Laser photobiomodulation of gene expression and release of growth factors and cytokines from cells in culture: a review of human and animal studies." *Photomed Laser Surg* 29 (5): 285-304. https://doi.org/10.1089/pho.2010.2846.

Perry, B. H., A. R. Sampson, B. H. Schwab, M. R. Karim, and J. M. Smiell. 2002. "A meta-analytic approach to an integrated summary of efficacy: a case study of becaplermin gel." *Control Clin Trials* 23 (4): 389-408. https://www.ncbi.nlm.nih.gov/pubmed/12161082.

Piccin, A., A. M. Di Pierro, L. Canzian, M. Primerano, D. Corvetta, G. Negri, G. Mazzoleni, G. Gastl, M. Steurer, I. Gentilini, K. Eisendle, and F. Fontanella. 2017. "Platelet gel: a new therapeutic tool with great potential." *Blood Transfus* 15 (4): 333-340. https://doi.org/10.2450/2016.0038-16.

Pierce, G. F., J. E. Tarpley, J. Tseng, J. Bready, D. Chang, W. C. Kenney, R. Rudolph, M. C. Robson, J. Vande Berg, P. Reid, S. Kaufman, C. L. Farrell. 1995. "Detection of platelet-derived growth factor (PDGF)-AA in actively healing human wounds treated with recombinant PDGF-BB and absence of PDGF in chronic nonhealing wounds." *J Clin Invest* 96 (3): 1336-50. https://doi.org/10.1172/JCI118169.

Pierce, G. F., J. E. Tarpley, R. M. Allman, P. S. Goode, C. M. Serdar, B. Morris, T. A. Mustoe, and J. Vande Berg. 1994. "Tissue repair processes in healing chronic pressure ulcers treated with recombinant platelet-derived growth factor BB." *Am J Pathol* 145 (6): 1399-410. https://www.ncbi.nlm.nih.gov/pubmed/7992843.

Plafki, C., P. Peters, M. Almeling, W. Welslau, and R. Busch. 2000. "Complications and side effects of hyperbaric oxygen therapy." *Aviat Space Environ Med* 71 (2): 119-24. https://www.ncbi.nlm.nih.gov/pubmed/10685584.

Priyadarshini, L.M.J., K.E.P. Babu, I.A. Thariq. 2018. "Effect of low-level laser therapy on diabetic foot ulcers: a randomized control trial." *Int Surg J.* 5(3): 1008-15. http://dx.doi.org/10.18203/2349-2902.isj20180821.

Prompers, L., M. Huijberts, J. Apelqvist, E. Jude, A. Piaggesi, K. Bakker, M. Edmonds, P. Holstein, A. Jirkovska, D. Mauricio, G. Ragnarson Tennvall, H. Reike, M. Spraul, L. Uccioli, V. Urbancic, K. Van Acker, J. van Baal, F. van Merode, and N. Schaper. 2007. "High prevalence of ischaemia, infection and serious comorbidity in patients with diabetic foot disease in Europe. Baseline results from the Eurodiale study." *Diabetologia* 50 (1): 18-25. https://doi.org/10.1007/s00125-006-0491-1.

Rac, M. W., L. G. Greer, and G. D. Wendel, Jr. 2010. "Jarisch-Herxheimer reaction triggered by group B *Streptococcus intrapartum* antibiotic prophylaxis." *Obstet Gynecol* 116 Suppl 2: 552-6. https://doi.org/10.1097/AOG.0b013e3181e7d065.

Ragnarson Tennvall, G., and J. Apelqvist. 2004. "Health-economic consequences of diabetic foot lesions." *Clin Infect Dis* 39 Suppl 2: S132-9. https://doi.org/10.1086/383275.

Rangaswamy, P., S. A. Rubby, and K. Prasanth. 2016. "Prospective study of platelet derived growth factor in wound healing of diabetic foot ulcers in indian population." *Int Surg J* 4 (1): 194–9. https://doi.org/10.18203/2349-2902.isj20164428.

Ravanti, L., and V. M. Kahari. 2000. "Matrix metalloproteinases in wound repair (review)." *Int J Mol Med* 6 (4): 391-407. https://www.ncbi.nlm.nih.gov/pubmed/10998429.

Redekop, W. K., J. McDonnell, P. Verboom, K. Lovas, and Z. Kalo. 2003. "The cost effectiveness of Apligraf treatment of diabetic foot ulcers." *Pharmacoeconomics* 21 (16): 1171-83. https://doi.org/10.2165/00019053-200321160-00003.

Rhoads, D. D., R. D. Wolcott, M. A. Kuskowski, B. M. Wolcott, L. S. Ward, and A. Sulakvelidze. 2009. "Bacteriophage therapy of venous leg ulcers in humans: results of a phase I safety trial." *J Wound Care* 18 (6): 237-8, 240-3. https://doi.org/10.12968/jowc.2009.18.6.42801.

Rice, J. B., U. Desai, A. K. Cummings, H. G. Birnbaum, M. Skornicki, and N. B. Parsons. 2014. "Burden of diabetic foot ulcers for medicare and private insurers." *Diabetes Care* 37 (3): 651-8. https://doi.org/10.2337/dc13-2176.

Richmond, N. A., A. C. Vivas, and R. S. Kirsner. 2013. "Topical and biologic therapies for diabetic foot ulcers." *Med Clin North Am* 97 (5): 883-98. https://doi.org/10.1016/j.mcna.2013.03.014.

Robson, M. C., L. G. Phillips, A. Thomason, B. W. Altrock, P. C. Pence, J. P. Heggers, A. F. Johnston, T. P. McHugh, M. S. Anthony, L. E. Robson, and et al. 1992. "Recombinant human platelet-derived growth factor-BB for the treatment of chronic pressure ulcers." *Ann Plast Surg* 29 (3): 193-201. https://www.ncbi.nlm.nih.gov/pubmed/1524367.

Robson, M. C., W. G. Payne, W. L. Garner, J. Biundo, V. F. Giacolone, D. M. Cooper, and P. Ouyang. 2005. "Intergrating the results of phase IV (post-marketing) clinical trial with four previous trials reinforces the position that Regranex (Becaplermin) Gel 0'. 01 is an effective adjunct to the treatment of diabetic foot ulcers" *J Appl Res* 5(1): 35–45. http://citeseerx.ist.psu.edu/viewdoc/summary?doi=10.1.1.418.6075.

Root, R. K., and D. C. Dale. 1999. "Granulocyte colony-stimulating factor and granulocyte-macrophage colony-stimulating factor: comparisons and potential for use in the treatment of infections in nonneutropenic patients." *J Infect Dis* 179 Suppl 2: S342-52. https://doi.org/10.1086/513857.

Rozman, P., and Z. Bolta. 2007. "Use of platelet growth factors in treating wounds and soft-tissue injuries." *Acta Dermatovenerol Alp Pannonica Adriat* 16 (4): 156-65. https://www.ncbi.nlm.nih.gov/pubmed/18204746.

Sabouri Ghannad, M., and A. Mohammadi. 2012. "Bacteriophage: time to re-evaluate the potential of phage therapy as a promising agent to control multidrug-resistant bacteria." *Iran J Basic Med Sci* 15 (2): 693-701. https://www.ncbi.nlm.nih.gov/pubmed/23494063.

Safavi, S. M., B. Kazemi, M. Esmaeili, A. Fallah, A. Modarresi, and M. Mir. 2008. "Effects of low-level He-Ne laser irradiation on the gene expression of IL-1beta, TNF-alpha, IFN-gamma, TGF-beta, bFGF, and PDGF in rat's gingiva." *Lasers Med Sci* 23 (3): 331-5. https://doi.org/10.1007/s10103-007-0491-5.

Saltmarche, A. E. 2008. "Low level laser therapy for healing acute and chronic wounds - the extendicare experience." *Int Wound J* 5 (2): 351-60. https://doi.org/10.1111/j.1742-481X.2008.00491.x.

Santema, K. T. B., R. M. Stoekenbroek, M. J. W. Koelemay, J. A. Reekers, L. M. C. van Dortmont, A. Oomen, L. Smeets, J. J. Wever, D. A. Legemate, D. T. Ubbink, and Damo Cles Study Group. 2018. "Hyperbaric Oxygen Therapy in the treatment of ischemic lower-extremity ulcers in patients with diabetes: results of the DAMO2CLES multicenter randomized clinical trial." *Diabetes Care* 41 (1): 112-119. https://doi.org/10.2337/dc17-0654.

Sari, Y., S. Saryono, E. Sutrisna, and H. Hartono. 2017. "A comparative study of the effects of vibration and electrical stimulation therapies on the acceleration of wound healing in diabetic ulcers." *Jurnal Ners* 12 (2): 253-60. https://doi.org/10.20473/jn.v12i2.4460.

Sato, N., K. Kashima, Y. Tanaka, H. Shimizu, and M. Mori. 1997. "Effect of granulocyte-colony stimulating factor on generation of oxygen-derived free radicals and myeloperoxidase activity in neutrophils from poorly controlled NIDDM patients." *Diabetes* 46 (1): 133-7. https://www.ncbi.nlm.nih.gov/pubmed/8971093.

Schindl, A., M. Schindl, H. Schon, R. Knobler, L. Havelec, and L. Schindl. 1998. "Low-intensity laser irradiation improves skin circulation in patients with diabetic microangiopathy." *Diabetes Care* 21 (4): 580-4. https://www.ncbi.nlm.nih.gov/pubmed/9571346.

Schintler, M. V. 2012. "Negative pressure therapy: theory and practice." *Diabetes Metab Res Rev* 28 Suppl 1: 72-7. https://doi.org/10.1002/dmrr.2243.

Sebastian, A., F. Syed, D. Perry, V. Balamurugan, J. Colthurst, I. H. Chaudhry, and A. Bayat. 2011. "Acceleration of cutaneous healing by electrical stimulation: degenerate electrical waveform down-regulates inflammation, up-regulates angiogenesis and advances remodeling in temporal punch biopsies in a human volunteer study." *Wound Repair Regen* 19 (6): 693-708. https://doi.org/10.1111/j.1524-475X.2011.00736.x.

Sepulveda, G., M. Espindola, M. Maureira, E. Sepulveda, J. Ignacio Fernandez, C. Oliva, A. Sanhueza, M. Vial, and C. Manterola. 2009. "[Negative-pressure wound therapy versus standard wound dressing in the treatment of diabetic foot amputation. A randomised controlled trial]." *Cir Esp* 86 (3): 171-7. https://doi.org/10.1016/j.ciresp.2009.03.020.

Shan, G. Q., Y. N. Zhang, J. Ma, Y. H. Li, D. M. Zuo, J. L. Qiu, B. Cheng, and Z. L. Chen. 2013. "Evaluation of the effects of homologous platelet gel on healing lower extremity wounds in patients with diabetes." *Int J Low Extrem Wounds* 12 (1): 22-9. https://doi.org/10.1177/1534734613477113.

Shen, G. Y., I. H. Park, Y. S. Song, H. W. Joo, Y. Lee, J. H. Shin, K. S. Kim, and H. Kim. 2016. "Local injection of granulocyte-colony

stimulating factor accelerates wound healing in a rat excisional wound model." *Tissue Eng Regen Med* 13 (3): 297-303. https://doi.org/10.1007/s13770-016-9054-9.
- Shimizu, N., M. Yamaguchi, T. Goseki, Y. Shibata, H. Takiguchi, T. Iwasawa, and Y. Abiko. 1995. "Inhibition of prostaglandin E2 and interleukin 1-beta production by low-power laser irradiation in stretched human periodontal ligament cells." *J Dent Res* 74 (7): 1382-8. https://doi.org/10.1177/00220345950740071001.
- Sibbald, R. G., P. Coutts, and K. Y. Woo. 2011. "Reduction of bacterial burden and pain in chronic wounds using a new polyhexamethylene biguanide antimicrobial foam dressing-clinical trial results." *Adv Skin Wound Care* 24 (2): 78-84. https://doi.org/10.1097/01.ASW.0000394027.82702.16.
- Siegbahn, A., A. Hammacher, B. Westermark, and C. H. Heldin. 1990. "Differential effects of the various isoforms of platelet-derived growth factor on chemotaxis of fibroblasts, monocytes, and granulocytes." *J Clin Invest* 85 (3): 916-20. https://doi.org/10.1172/JCI114519.
- Singer, A. J., and R. A. Clark. 1999. "Cutaneous wound healing." *N Engl J Med* 341 (10): 738-46. https://doi.org/10.1056/NEJM199909023411006.
- Slopek, S., A. Kucharewicz-Krukowska, B. Weber-Dabrowska, and M. Dabrowski. 1985a. "Results of bacteriophage treatment of suppurative bacterial infections. IV. Evaluation of the results obtained in 370 cases." *Arch Immunol Ther Exp (Warsz)* 33 (2): 219-40. https://www.ncbi.nlm.nih.gov/pubmed/2935115.
- Slopek, S., A. Kucharewicz-Krukowska, B. Weber-Dabrowska, and M. Dabrowski. 1985b. "Results of bacteriophage treatment of suppurative bacterial infections. V. Evaluation of the results obtained in children." *Arch Immunol Ther Exp (Warsz)* 33 (2): 241-59. https://www.ncbi.nlm.nih.gov/pubmed/2935116.
- Slopek, S., A. Kucharewicz-Krukowska, B. Weber-Dabrowska, and M. Dabrowski. 1985c. "Results of bacteriophage treatment of suppurative bacterial infections. VI. Analysis of treatment of suppurative

staphylococcal infections." *Arch Immunol Ther Exp (Warsz)* 33 (2): 261-73. https://www.ncbi.nlm.nih.gov/pubmed/2935117.

Slopek, S., B. Weber-Dabrowska, M. Dabrowski, and A. Kucharewicz-Krukowska. 1987. "Results of bacteriophage treatment of suppurative bacterial infections in the years 1981-1986." *Arch Immunol Ther Exp (Warsz)* 35 (5): 569-83. https://www.ncbi.nlm.nih.gov/pubmed/3455647.

Slopek, S., I. Durlakowa, B. Weber-Dabrowska, A. Kucharewicz-Krukowska, M. Dabrowski, and R. Bisikiewicz. 1983a. "Results of bacteriophage treatment of suppurative bacterial infections. I. General evaluation of the results." *Arch Immunol Ther Exp (Warsz)* 31 (3): 267-91. https://www.ncbi.nlm.nih.gov/pubmed/6651484.

Slopek, S., I. Durlakowa, B. Weber-Dabrowska, A. Kucharewicz-Krukowska, M. Dabrowski, and R. Bisikiewicz. 1983b. "Results of bacteriophage treatment of suppurative bacterial infections. II. Detailed evaluation of the results." *Arch Immunol Ther Exp (Warsz)* 31 (3): 293-327. https://www.ncbi.nlm.nih.gov/pubmed/6651485.

Slopek, S., I. Durlakowa, B. Weber-Dabrowska, M. Dabrowski, and A. Kucharewicz-Krukowska. 1984. "Results of bacteriophage treatment of suppurative bacterial infections. III. Detailed evaluation of the results obtained in further 150 cases." *Arch Immunol Ther Exp (Warsz)* 32 (3): 317-35. https://www.ncbi.nlm.nih.gov/pubmed/6395825.

Smith, H. W., M. B. Huggins, and K. M. Shaw. 1987. "The control of experimental Escherichia coli diarrhoea in calves by means of bacteriophages." *J Gen Microbiol* 133 (5): 1111-26. https://doi.org/10.1099/00221287-133-5-1111.

Snyder, D. L., N. Sullivan, and K. M. Schoelles. 2012. *Skin Substitutes for Treating Chronic Wounds*, AHRQ Technology Assessments. Rockville (MD).

Solis, L. R., S. Gyawali, P. Seres, C. A. Curtis, S. L. Chong, R. B. Thompson, and V. K. Mushahwar. 2011. "Effects of intermittent electrical stimulation on superficial pressure, tissue oxygenation, and discomfort levels for the prevention of deep tissue injury." *Ann Biomed Eng* 39 (2): 649-63. https://doi.org/10.1007/s10439-010-0193-1.

Sridharan, K., and G. Sivaramakrishnan. 2018. "Growth factors for diabetic foot ulcers: mixed treatment comparison analysis of randomized clinical trials." *Br J Clin Pharmacol* 84 (3): 434-444. https://doi.org/10.1111/bcp.13470.

Steed, D. L. 1995. "Clinical evaluation of recombinant human platelet-derived growth factor for the treatment of lower extremity diabetic ulcers. Diabetic Ulcer Study Group." *J Vasc Surg* 21 (1): 71-8; discussion 79-81. https://www.ncbi.nlm.nih.gov/pubmed/7823364.

Steed, D. L., C. Attinger, T. Colaizzi, M. Crossland, M. Franz, L. Harkless, A. Johnson, H. Moosa, M. Robson, T. Serena, P. Sheehan, A. Veves, and L. Wiersma-Bryant. 2006. "Guidelines for the treatment of diabetic ulcers." *Wound Repair Regen* 14 (6): 680-92. https://doi.org/10.1111/j.1524-475X.2006.00176.x.

Stern, A., and R. Sorek. 2011. "The phage-host arms race: shaping the evolution of microbes." *Bioessays* 33 (1): 43-51. https://doi.org/10.1002/bies.201000071.

Strauss, M. B. 2005. "Hyperbaric oxygen as an intervention for managing wound hypoxia: its role and usefulness in diabetic foot wounds." *Foot Ankle Int* 26 (1): 15-8. https://www.ncbi.nlm.nih.gov/pubmed/15680113.

Sulakvelidze, A. 2011. "Bacteriophage: A new journal for the most ubiquitous organisms on Earth." *Bacteriophage* 1 (1): 1-2. https://doi.org/10.4161/bact.1.1.15030.

Taha, O. A., P. L. Connerton, I. F. Connerton, and A. El-Shibiny. 2018. "Bacteriophage ZCKP1: a potential treatment for *Klebsiella pneumoniae* isolated from diabetic foot patients." *Front Microbiol* 9: 2127. https://doi.org/10.3389/fmicb.2018.02127.

Tanaka, T., N. Panthee, Y. Itoda, N. Yamauchi, M. Fukayama, and M. Ono. 2016. "Negative pressure wound therapy induces early wound healing by increased and accelerated expression of vascular endothelial growth factor receptors." *Eur J Plast Surg* 39: 247-256. https://doi.org/10.1007/s00238-016-1200-z.

Tascini, C., A. Piaggesi, E. Tagliaferri, E. Iacopi, S. Fondelli, A. Tedeschi, L. Rizzo, A. Leonildi, and F. Menichetti. 2011. "Microbiology at first visit of moderate-to-severe diabetic foot infection with antimicrobial activity and a survey of quinolone monotherapy." *Diabetes Res Clin Pract* 94 (1): 133-9. https://doi.org/10.1016/j.diabres.2011.07.017.

Tchanque-Fossuo, C. N., D. Ho, S. E. Dahle, E. Koo, C. S. Li, R. R. Isseroff, and J. Jagdeo. 2016. "A systematic review of low-level light therapy for treatment of diabetic foot ulcer." *Wound Repair Regen* 24 (2): 418-26. https://doi.org/10.1111/wrr.12399.

Thackham, J. A., D. L. McElwain, and R. J. Long. 2008. "The use of hyperbaric oxygen therapy to treat chronic wounds: A review." *Wound Repair Regen* 16 (3): 321-30. https://doi.org/10.1111/j.1524-475X.2008.00372.x.

Thakral, G., J. Lafontaine, B. Najafi, T. K. Talal, P. Kim, and L. A. Lavery. 2013. "Electrical stimulation to accelerate wound healing." *Diabet Foot Ankle* 4. https://doi.org/10.3402/dfa.v4i0.22081.

To, E., R. Dyck, S. Gerber, S. Kadavil, and K. Y. Woo. 2016. "The Effectiveness of Topical Polyhexamethylene Biguanide (PHMB) Agents for the Treatment of Chronic Wounds: A Systematic Review." *Surg Technol Int* 29: 45-51. https://www.ncbi.nlm.nih.gov/pubmed/27608742.

Tonnesen, M. G., X. Feng, and R. A. Clark. 2000. "Angiogenesis in wound healing." *J Investig Dermatol Symp Proc* 5 (1): 40-6. https://doi.org/10.1046/j.1087-0024.2000.00014.x.

Torkaman, G. 2014. "Electrical stimulation of wound healing: a review of animal experimental evidence." *Adv Wound Care (New Rochelle)* 3 (2): 202-218. https://doi.org/10.1089/wound.2012.0409.

Tzeng, D. Y., T. F. Deuel, J. S. Huang, and R. L. Baehner. 1985. "Platelet-derived growth factor promotes human peripheral monocyte activation." *Blood* 66 (1): 179-83. https://www.ncbi.nlm.nih.gov/pubmed/2988667.

Ud-Din, S., A. Sebastian, P. Giddings, J. Colthurst, S. Whiteside, J. Morris, R. Nuccitelli, C. Pullar, M. Baguneid, and A. Bayat. 2015. "Angiogenesis is induced and wound size is reduced by electrical stimulation in an acute wound healing model in human skin." *PLoS One* 10 (4): e0124502. https://doi.org/10.1371/journal.pone.0124502.

van Battum, P., N. Schaper, L. Prompers, J. Apelqvist, E. Jude, A. Piaggesi, K. Bakker, M. Edmonds, P. Holstein, A. Jirkovska, D. Mauricio, G. Ragnarson Tennvall, H. Reike, M. Spraul, L. Uccioli, V. Urbancic, K. van Acker, J. van Baal, I. Ferreira, and M. Huijberts. 2011. "Differences in minor amputation rate in diabetic foot disease throughout Europe are in part explained by differences in disease severity at presentation." *Diabet Med* 28 (2): 199-205. https://doi.org/10.1111/j.1464-5491.2010.03192.x.

Velnar, T., T. Bailey, and V. Smrkolj. 2009. "The wound healing process: an overview of the cellular and molecular mechanisms." *J Int Med Res* 37 (5): 1528-42. https://doi.org/10.1177/147323000903700531.

Veves, A., V. Falanga, D. G. Armstrong, M. L. Sabolinski, and Study Apligraf Diabetic Foot Ulcer. 2001. "Graftskin, a human skin equivalent, is effective in the management of noninfected neuropathic diabetic foot ulcers: a prospective randomized multicenter clinical trial." *Diabetes Care* 24 (2): 290-5. https://www.ncbi.nlm.nih.gov/pubmed/11213881.

Wagner, F. W., Jr. 1981. "The dysvascular foot: a system for diagnosis and treatment." *Foot Ankle* 2 (2): 64-122. https://www.ncbi.nlm.nih.gov/pubmed/7319435.

Wang, T., R. He, J. Zhao, J. C. Mei, M. Z. Shao, Y. Pan, J. Zhang, H. S. Wu, M. Yu, W. C. Yan, L. M. Liu, F. Liu, and W. P. Jia. 2017. "Negative pressure wound therapy inhibits inflammation and upregulates activating transcription factor-3 and downregulates nuclear factor-kappaB in diabetic patients with foot ulcerations." *Diabetes Metab Res Rev* 33 (4). https://doi.org/10.1002/dmrr.2871.

Wang, T., X. Li, L. Fan, B. Chen, J. Liu, Y. Tao, and X. Wang. 2019. "Negative pressure wound therapy promoted wound healing by suppressing inflammation via down-regulating MAPK-JNK signaling pathway in diabetic foot patients." *Diabetes Res Clin Pract* 150: 81-89. https://doi.org/10.1016/j.diabres.2019.02.024.

Waycaster, C. R., A. M. Gilligan, and T. A. Motley. 2016. "Cost-effectiveness of Becaplermin Gel on diabetic foot ulcer healing

changes in wound surface area." *J Am Podiatr Med Assoc* 106 (4): 273-82. https://doi.org/10.7547/15-004.
Werner, S., and R. Grose. 2003. "Regulation of wound healing by growth factors and cytokines." *Physiol Rev* 83 (3): 835-70. https://doi.org/10.1152/physrev.2003.83.3.835.
Widgerow, A. D. 2014. "Bioengineered skin substitute considerations in the diabetic foot ulcer." *Ann Plast Surg* 73 (2): 239-44. https://doi.org/10.1097/SAP.0b013e31826eac22.
Wieman, T. J., J. M. Smiell, and Y. Su. 1998. "Efficacy and safety of a topical gel formulation of recombinant human platelet-derived growth factor-BB (becaplermin) in patients with chronic neuropathic diabetic ulcers. A phase III randomized placebo-controlled double-blind study." *Diabetes Care* 21 (5): 822-7. https://www.ncbi.nlm.nih.gov/pubmed/9589248.
Wild, S., G. Roglic, A. Green, R. Sicree, and H. King. 2004. "Global prevalence of diabetes: estimates for the year 2000 and projections for 2030." *Diabetes Care* 27 (5): 1047-53. https://www.ncbi.nlm.nih.gov/pubmed/15111519.
Wilson, J. R., J. G. Mills, I. D. Prather, and S. D. Dimitrijevich. 2005. "A toxicity index of skin and wound cleansers used on *in vitro* fibroblasts and keratinocytes." *Adv Skin Wound Care* 18 (7): 373-8. https://www.ncbi.nlm.nih.gov/pubmed/16160464.
Wirsing, P. G., A. D. Habrom, T. M. Zehnder, S. Friedli, and M. Blatti. 2015. "Wireless micro current stimulation--an innovative electrical stimulation method for the treatment of patients with leg and diabetic foot ulcers." *Int Wound J* 12 (6): 693-8. https://doi.org/10.1111/iwj.12204.
Wittebole, X., S. De Roock, and S. M. Opal. 2014. "A historical overview of bacteriophage therapy as an alternative to antibiotics for the treatment of bacterial pathogens." *Virulence* 5 (1): 226-35. https://doi.org/10.4161/viru.25991.
World Health Organization. 2016. *Global report on diabetes*. Switzerland: WHO Press.

Wu, Q. 2018. "Hyperbaric oxygen for treatment of diabetic foot ulcers: love you more than I can say." *Ann Transl Med* 6 (11): 228. https://doi.org/10.21037/atm.2018.04.33.

Wu, S. C., W. Marston, and D. G. Armstrong. 2010. "Wound care: the role of advanced wound healing technologies." *J Vasc Surg* 52 (3 Suppl): 59S-66S. https://doi.org/10.1016/j.jvs.2010.06.009.

Wunderlich, R. P., E. J. Peters, and L. A. Lavery. 2000. "Systemic hyperbaric oxygen therapy: lower-extremity wound healing and the diabetic foot." *Diabetes Care* 23 (10): 1551-5. https://www.ncbi.nlm.nih.gov/pubmed/11023151.

Wynn, M., and S. Freeman. 2019. "The efficacy of negative pressure wound therapy for diabetic foot ulcers: A systematised review." *J Tissue Viability*. https://doi.org/10.1016/j.jtv.2019.04.001.

Xu, S. M., and T. Liang. 2016. "Clinical observation of the application of autologous peripheral blood stem cell transplantation for the treatment of diabetic foot gangrene." *Exp Ther Med* 11 (1): 283-288. https://doi.org/10.3892/etm.2015.2888.

Yazdanpanah, L., M. Nasiri, and S. Adarvishi. 2015. "Literature review on the management of diabetic foot ulcer." *World J Diabetes* 6 (1): 37-53. https://doi.org/10.4239/wjd.v6.i1.37.

Zaulyanov, L., and R. S. Kirsner. 2007. "A review of a bi-layered living cell treatment (Apligraf) in the treatment of venous leg ulcers and diabetic foot ulcers." *Clin Interv Aging* 2 (1): 93-8. https://www.ncbi.nlm.nih.gov/pubmed/18044080.

Zhao, D., S. Luo, W. Xu, J. Hu, S. Lin, and N. Wang. 2017. "Efficacy and safety of Hyperbaric Oxygen Therapy used in patients with diabetic foot: a meta-analysis of randomized clinical trials." *Clin Ther* 39 (10): 2088-2094 e2. https://doi.org/10.1016/j.clinthera.2017.08.014.

Zhao, M. 2009. "Electrical fields in wound healing - an overriding signal that directs cell migration." *Semin Cell Dev Biol* 20 (6): 674-82. https://doi.org/10.1016/j.semcdb.2008.12.009.

Zhao, M., B. Song, J. Pu, T. Wada, B. Reid, G. Tai, F. Wang, A. Guo, P. Walczysko, Y. Gu, T. Sasaki, A. Suzuki, J. V. Forrester, H. R. Bourne, P. N. Devreotes, C. D. McCaig, and J. M. Penninger. 2006. "Electrical signals control wound healing through phosphatidylinositol-3-OH kinase-gamma and PTEN." *Nature* 442 (7101): 457-60. https://doi.org/10.1038/nature04925.

Ziyadeh, N., D. Fife, A. M. Walker, G. S. Wilkinson, and J. D. Seeger. 2011. "A matched cohort study of the risk of cancer in users of becaplermin." *Adv Skin Wound Care* 24 (1): 31-9. https://doi.org/10.1097/01.ASW.0000392922.30229.b3.

Chapter 5

THE EFFECTS OF SOCIAL SUPPORT AND HOPE IN THE HEALING OF DIABETIC FOOT ULCERS TREATED WITH STANDARD CARE

Ayfer Peker Karatoprak[1,*] *and Süreyya Karaöz*[2]

[1]Health Care Services- Podology,
Kocaeli University, Kocaeli, Turkey
[2]Faculty of Health Sciences, İstanbul Bilgi University,
İstanbul, Turkey

ABSTRACT

Aim: This study was carried out to investigate the effects of "Social Support" and "Hope" on 50% reduction of wound size after four weeks of treatment with standard care in patients with Grade B, Stage I diabetic foot ulcer.

Methods: The study population was composed of patients with Grade B, Stage I diabetic foot ulcers. The *study sample included 34 patients,*

---

[*] Corresponding Author's E-mail: pekayfer@gmail.com.

aged ≥40 years, with type 2 diabetes, HbA1c concentration of >7%. This *study used four data collection tools including* two *questionnaire and Beck Hopelessness Scale (BHS); Multidimensional Scale of Perceived Social Support (MSPSS).* All *patients received evidence-based standard* care. W*ound surface area was measured at days* 1 and 30 to determine whether 50% percent decrease has been achieved. T *test, correlation analysis, and chi-square test were used for data analysis.*

Findings: A *positive correlation was found between* family social support and healing percentage (r = 406, p = 0.01). A*ccording to BHS,* patients with wounds healed over 50% in size had mild, and those with wounds healed less than 50% had moderate scores. There was a *negative correlation between social support and hopelessness* (r =-449, p = 0.01). A *negative correlation was found with social support from the family* (r = -539, p = 0.01) and *the friends* (r = -457, p = 0.01), and hopelessness.

Conclusion: Social support and high motivation had a positive effect on wound healing in patients with diabetic foot ulcers. Family social support *affects healing in a positive way, but hopelessness in a negative way.*

1. INTRODUCTION

Diabetes mellitus is a common metabolic disorder that can cause various complications [1, 2]. According to the studies, the prevalence of diabetes is rapidly increasing both in Turkey and in the world [1, 3]. It is an important health issue for the high healthcare costs and serious complications that may involve the patients with different aspects [1].

Diabetic foot ulcer is a major complication of diabetes mellitus. The diabetic foot ulcer, although highly preventable, has become a mental, physical, social, and economic burden affecting the patients [4, 5]. A common manifestation of the diabetic complications is the diabetic foot ulcer, and it significantly affects the quality of life of the patients. Diabetic foot ulcer causes various degrees of dependency in activity, inability, negative affectivity, and labour loss. Besides, longer bed occupancy and higher healthcare costs, diabetic foot ulcer also increases the risk of lower limb amputation and mortality [1, 6]. Almost 12-25% of diabetic patients will be suffering from diabetic foot ulcer during their lifetime, and 10-15% of patients admitted with diabetic foot requiring surgical intervention [7, 8,

9]. The amputation rate in diabetic foot disease throughout Europe was reported as 0.5-0.8% [10]. In the United States, 85% of lower-extremity amputations are preceded by foot ulcers in patients with diabetes mellitus [11].

Although wound care is an important aspect in diabetic foot ulcer management, other factors, such as the patient's emotional state, hope, life commitment, social support resources, and patient compliance to the treatment should be considered in its management [12, 13, 14, 15]. The treatment and care of the diabetics require a multidisciplinary approach because of the extensive nature of the problem. The main objective of a healthcare team in the management of a diabetic patient is to achieve metabolic control with emphasis on health education, and to improve survival and quality of life. As a key member of the healthcare team, the nurse has an important role to play in educating the patient, improving patient self-care skills, and providing adequate care.

1.1. Limitations of the Study

The definite population size is not known; lack of a random sampling technique and a small sample size is a limitation of the current study. Financial constraints is one of the factors limited our sample size.

1.1.1. Aim

This study was designed to investigate the effects of "social support" and "hope" on 50% reduction of wound size after four weeks of treatment with standard care in patients who presented Diabetic Foot/Podology Clinic of a university hospital, with Grade B, Stage I diabetic foot ulcer.

1.2. Methods

1.2.1. Type of the Study

This is a cohort study.

1.2.2. Study Sample

Diabetic Foot/Podology Clinic of Kocaeli University Research and Training Hospital has recently been founded, the sample size was estimated via the formula described by Karasar [16] for cases when the population was not known, as 34 patients. The sample size was determined by considering the factors involved in wound healing. The study sample was consisted of patients aged ≥40 years, with type 2 diabetes, HbA1c concentration of >7%, and Grade B, Stage I diabetic foot ulcers according to University of Texas, San Antonio, Diabetic Wound Classification system (Table 2.1). Patients with known risk factors affecting wound healing, autoimmune diseases, malnutrition, an ankle-brachial index less than 0.9, major operation in the last 3 months, psychological or physical trauma during the study period, and those taking corticosteroids or immunosuppressive therapy were excluded from the study. Also, the wounds secondary to burn injury were not included. All the patients admitted to the Diabetic Foot/Podology Clinic of Kocaeli University Research and Training Hospital since the onset of the study and met the patient selection criteria were enrolled in the trial. Recruitment was terminated when estimated sample size (34 patients) was reached.

1.2.3. Data Collection

Four data collection tools including a questionnaire on demographic characteristics and factors affecting wound healing; another questionnaire on wound assessment and follow-up via physical examination; Beck Hopelessness Scale (BHS), and Multidimensional Scale of Perceived Social Support (MSPSS) were used in this study. The population in which the data of the study were obtained consisted of patients who agreed to participate in the study, and who were followed-up for Grade B, Stage I diabetic foot ulcers classified according to Diabetic Wound Classification system described by University of Texas, San Antonio. Fifty percent decrease in any wound size was considered as reliable information about the healing potential [17, 18]. Considering the phases of wound healing, 25-30 days (4 weeks) was considered sufficient time to assess healing.

All patients received standard care according to a diabetic foot ulcer study protocol developed by the researcher based on published guidelines. The researcher was trained for four months in Steno Diabetes Center and Copenhagen School of Podiatry in management and care of diabetic foot ulcers. The headlines of the training included standard care, determination of localisation and depth of ulcer, assessment of infection, reducing the pressure, repair of skin perfusion, treatment of infection, metabolic control, treatment of comorbidities, local wound care, education of patients and family members, and identification of the reasons, and prevention of recurrences [19, 20, 21, 22]. Patients have been evaluated for conditions such as hyperglycemia, peripheral vascular disease, infection, and charcot joints. Patients with hyperglycemia were referred to an endocrinologist, those with peripheral vascular disease to a vascular surgeon, those with signs of infection to an infectious diseases specialist, and patients with suspected Charcot joints to an orthopedician. Patients with impaired skin perfusion were not included in the study.

In the first evaluation visit, foot examination was performed; each wound size was measured and recorded on the wound assessment and follow-up form; the sociodemographic characteristics and the factors affecting wound healing were recorded; and BHS and MSPSS were applied to each patient. The patients were informed about the prevention and treatment of diabetic foot ulcers and were given a training book, prepared by the researcher, containing recommendations that the patient with diabetic foot ulcer should follow. The patients were supervised to perform active and passive exercises according to the localization of their wound(s) and immobilization status of the patient. All patients continued to be informed about the prevention and treatment of diabetic foot ulcers in the following three visits.

Wound healing was evaluated in each patient for one month. Wound surface area (cm^2) was calculated on days 1, 8, 15, 22 and 30; status of the wound, dressing-related problems, and training applied to patients were also recorded. It was calculated whether there was 50% reduction in wound surface area on days 1 and 30. BHS and MSPSS scores were compared between patients with or without 50% reduction after 4 weeks.

Gender, body mass index (BMI), insulin use status, etiology of diabetic foot ulcer(s), ulcer size, duration, depth and severity of the ulcer(s), duration of diabetes, body temperature, blood pressure, hematocrit level, blood albumin level, presence of chronic disease other than diabetes (i.e., congestive heart failure, chronic liver disease, peripheral vascular disease, hypertension), foot deformities, neuropathy,, and vascular failure, and alcohol and smoking habits were considered as factors affecting to achieve a 50% reduction after 4 weeks.

1.2.4. Data Analysis

The data were analyzed using Statistical Package for the Social Sciences (SPSS) computer software version 15.0. The statistical analysis of data by Kolmogorov-Smirnov test showed normal distribution ($p > 0.05$). Chi-square test, Fisher's exact chi-square test, the difference between two means test, and correlation analysis were used for the analysis. Non-parametric tests were used when assumptions of parametric tests were not met. Yates' correction was used when the number of observed data was less than 5, and for discrete data.

1.2.5. The Ethical Aspects of the Study

Approval was obtained for the title and content of the study protocol from Kocaeli University Institute of Health Sciences and Kocaeli University Human Research Ethics Committee before the study was carried out. Before any study-related procedures, patients were informed about the purpose, duration and design of the study, and their verbal and written consent was obtained.

2. RESULTS

2.1. Sociodemographic and Disease-Related Characteristics of Patients

Fifty-two percent of the patients were ≥61 year-old, 88.2% were married, 82.4% had primary school education, and 100% were under social security coverage. Most of the patients did not have a smoking habit, and none of them consumed alcohol (91.2%, 100%). Regarding physical exercise, 79.4% of the patients did not practice regular exercise. Further, 52.9% of the patients were not monitored by a doctor regularly for their diabetes, 58.8% had difficulties to access healthcare services, and 5.2% reported lack of confidence about healthcare providers

A total of 85.3% of the patients were being treated with oral antidiabetic drugs and insulin, 55.9% did not participate in diabetes educations, 58.9% believed that they did not actually benefit from diabetes education, 64.7% had an ulcer on the front part of the foot, 64.7% had only one ulcer, 55.9% did not have a history of diabetic foot disease, 58.8% did not have a prior history of amputation related to diabetes, and 67.6% received foot examination related to diabetes.

2.2. Social Support

The scores of MSPSS were higher in patients with over 50% reduction in wound size than those with less than 50% reduction after four weeks of treatment (Mann-Whitney U Test, p = 0.001). Subgroup analysis of MSPSS showed that family social support scores of the patients with wounds healed above 50% was higher than that of those with wounds healed below 50% (Mann-Whitney U Test, p = 0.001) (Table 1).

Table 1. Recovery of patients according to their social support scores

Social support	Median (25-75) value in recovered patients (n = 18)	Median (25-75) value in unrecovered patients (n = 16)	P value
Total social support scores	79 (76-84)	71 (66-78)	0.001
Family social support scores	28 (28-28)	22 (18-25)	0.001
Friend social support scores	26 (20-28)	25 (20-28)	0.53
Significant other social support scores	28 (26-28)	26 (24-28)	0.11

A positive correlation was noted between family social support and the percentage of recovery (r = 406, p = 0.01), and the rate of recovery increased with increased family social support (Table 2).

Table 2. The relationship between perceived social support and recovery

Perceived social support	Percentage of Recovery	
	r	p
Family social support	0.406	0.01
Friend social support	0.194	0.09
Significant others social support	0.256	0.32
Total score of social support	0.314	0.22

2.3. Hopelessness

The median score on the BHS was 5 in patients with over 50% reduction in wound size after four weeks of treatment, and 9 in patients with less than 50% reduction. Although the difference was not statistically significant, patients with over 50% reduction in wound size had low levels of hopelessness, and those with less than 50% reduction in wound size had moderate levels of hopelessness.

Table 3. Recovery of patients according to their hopelessness scores (Median)

Hopelessness	Median (25-75) value in recovered patients (n = 18)	Median (25-75) value in unrecovered patients (n = 16)	P value
Hopelessness score	5 (3-10.75)	9 (3.25-14.75)	0.34
Feelings about future	2 (1-4)	3 (1.2-4)	0.38
Loss of motivation	1 (1-2)	2 (1-5)	0.03
Expectations about future	2 (1-5)	2 (1-5)	0.97

Subgroup analysis of BHS showed that self-perceived motivation loss scores of the patients with over 50% reduction in wound size was lower than that of those with less than 50% reduction in wound size (Mann-Whitney U Test, p = 0.03) (Table 3).

2.4. The Relationship between Social Support and Hopelessness

A negative correlation was found between social support from the family and hopelessness (r = -0.539, p = 0.01). However, no significant relationship was observed between social support from friends and hopelessness (r = -0.223, p = 0.22). A negative association was found between social support from significant others and hopelessness (r = -0.457, p = 0.01). Furthermore, a negative relationship was detected between total score of social support and hopelessness score (r = -0.449, p = 0.01).

Table 4. The relationship between perceived social support and hopelessness (n = 34)

Perceived social support	Hopelessness	
	r	p
Family social support	-0.539	0.01
Friend social support	-0.223	0.22
Significant other social support	-0.457	0.01
Total score of social support	-0.449	0.01

3. DISCUSSION

The wound healing is a natural process that depends on many factors. Recently, not only physiological but also psychological causes of diabetes and its complications have been investigated. Psychosocial factors contribute to the development of complications related to diabetes as well as the healing process in either a positive or negative way. Diabetic foot ulcers, one of the major complications of diabetes mellitus, have both physiological and psychological effects. Diabetic foot ulcers negatively affect patient's quality of life, and also cause various degrees of dependency in physical activity, inability, negative affectivity, and need of support from social environment. The treatment and care require a multidisciplinary assessment and approach because of the multiple needs and requirements of the diabetic foot ulcer problem [23, 24, 25, 26]. In this study, the effects of social support and hope were investigated in patients treated with evidence based standard care.

Our study results revealed a positive correlation between family social support and recovery, and the more extensive famiiy support was perceived to be, the better the healing process could take place. Recovery declines with high level of hopelessness, and loss of motivation negatively affects recovery. Patients with wounds healed over 50% had mild, and those with wounds healed less than 50% had moderate hopelessness scores. Although the difference was not statistically significant, the scores of hopelessness for the feelings and expectations about future were higher in patients with less than 50% reduction in wound size than those with 50% reduction. Loss of motivation was more pronounced in patients with poor recovery. In addition, a negative correlation was found between social support and hopelessness, and hopelessness decreased with the increase of social support level.

Many studies have been conducted to investigate the psychosocial factors affecting the development of diabetes and its complications, but the effects of social support and hope on the healing of diabetic foot ulcers have not been examined. The studies revealed that psychosocial factors were involved in the development of diabetes complications. Also, diabetes itself may induce psychosocial problems [27]. Social support plays a major role in coping with stress, and protects people against stressful life events and harmful effects of stress [28]. Proper social support ultimately results in individual physical health and psychological well-being, and is positively correlated with sense of belonging, self-confidence and self-esteem [29, 30, 31]. Results indicated that patients who perceived higher levels of social support were more likely to have a higher level of self-care [32, 33]; also, social networks may have negative influences on patien's self-care [33]. In our study, it was found that social support had a positive effect on healing in diabetic foot ulcers. Social support plays an important role in management and care process of diabetic foot ulcers. Moreover, social support is important in the prevention as well as the treatment of complications in diabetic patients. Patients need the help of family members at home care, and also to reach out to health care providers. Social support not only protects people against stressful life events and harmful effects of stress, but also increases treatment compliance and quality of care.

There are studies that have shown that negative affectivity increased associated with diabetes. Stress is the most common negative feeling, followed by anxiety, discomfort, nervousness and hopelessness in patients with diabetes mellitus [34, 35]. Many researchs showed that hopelessness increases the risk of complications, and negatively affects quality of care [36, 37]. There are many factors that lead to hopelessness during disease process, including lack of sufficient social support. Hopelessness is a proximal cause of depression and thought of suicide (38); furthermore, depression/anxiety reduce quality of life and has positive effect on peripheral neuropathy [39]. To have a chronic disease may also be associated with negative affectivity. Feelings of weakness and despair have been shown to increase in patients with chronic nonhealing wounds such as venous leg ulcers and diabetic ulcers [40]. The relationship between hope and immune system function was stated, and nowadays the relationship between wound healing and psychological factors has attracted increasing interest. Although the mechanisms underlying these interactions are not understood, the literature demonstrates that psychological stress negatively affects immune function and wound healing [41]. Prevention of health problems caused by negative affectivity is as important as prevention of negative affectivity caused by health problems. Studies have also shown that negative affectivity increases complications, adversely affects self-care behaviors, and decreases quality of life. According to results of our study, negative affectivity adversely affects recovery.

There is a positive correlation between social support and hope. In our study, the rate of improvement was not similar among patients with similar physiological characteristics and treated with standard care. Fifty three percent of our patients initially treated with standard care subsequently showed 50% reduction in wound size whereas the remaining 47% did not. According to the results of our study, level of hopelessness is inversely correlated with recovery, while loss of motivation adversely and social support positively affected recovery. Moreover, social support adversely affected hopelessness, and as social support increased, hopelessness decreased. Our results suggest that, the assessment of physiological factors is as important as the assessment of social and psychological factors. Family members or friends give hope and courage to patients, and make contributions to combat their disease [42]. Family support is known to be an especially important factor for chronic diseased patients. A study of hemodialysis patients showed that negative life events and lack of social support led to hopelessness [43], and a negative correlation was observed between perceived family social support level and hopelessness [44]. In some studies low or lack of family support has been linked to early mortality and elevated risk for suicide [45, 46], while other studies showed a positive effect of family support on psychological well-being and survival [47, 48]. In our study, a negative correlation was found between social support from family and significant others and hopelessness, and as social support increases hopelessness level decreased. The loving support from surroundings helps to alleviate concerns about the future and relieves pessimism and despair. Hopelessness leads to poor compliance with treatment. However, the key to regaining of patient's former life energy is by being hopeful and optimistic. This study demonstrates the importance of support provided by healthcare professionals to diabetic patients who live alone. The nurse plays a key role in providing this support and in fostering communication between family members and patient. Patients with inadequate social support should have an easy access to the nurses and easily seek support.

In our study, the groups were matched for all physiological parameters that can affect wound healing, and the patients with systemic problems that impair wound healing were excluded from the study. When we investigated the relationship between physiological parameters and healing of diabetic foot ulcers, we found that high blood pressure and history of diabetic foot complication adversely affected wound healing. Our findings in this research are consistent with studies in the literature; history of diabetic foot complication is one of the factors that impair wound healing [22], and high blood pressure may significantly increase risk of cardiovascular complications in diabetic patients. A significant difference was not observed between the groups on other factors, and this also supports our findings.

Diabetic foot ulcer is a preventable complication of diabetes. Evidence-based guidelines for the management of diabetic foot problems note that diabetic foot ulcers can be prevented to a great extent by regular foot examinations and proper therapeutic measures. Therefore, regular diabetic neuropathy assessment, vascular assessment, joint and muscle examination, and walking analysis are recommended. Care of the pressure points on the plantar aspect of the foot is essential to prevent diabetic foot ulcers [1, 10]. In our study, insoles, manufactured according to pedography analysis, were used. During this analysis, the pressure points in the patient's feet are detected; the patient may then be treated to prevent the development of ulcer. Also the pressure is evenly distributed across the foot and heel. Proper off-loading is essential for the healing of diabetic foot ulcers. Abnormal pressure can be distributed by insoles to prevent recurrence. For these reasons, it is essential to establish qualified diabetic foot clinics all over the country, to standardize care, and to improve the standard of nursery education for the prevention and treatment of diabetic foot ulcers.

CONCLUSION AND RECOMMENDATIONS

Conclusion

In our study, we have detected the effects of social support and hope on the healing of diabetic foot ulcer in patients who received standard care.

According to the results of our study,

- level of hopelessness was inversely correlated with the healing of diabetic foot ulcers, and loss of motivation adversely affected recovery;
- patients with wounds healed 50% had mild, and those with wounds healed less than 50% had moderate hopelessness scores after four weeks of treatment;
- although the difference was not statistically significant, the scores of hopelessness for the feelings and expectations about future were higher in patients with less than 50% reduction in wound size than those with 50% reduction;
- loss of motivation was more pronounced in patients with poor recovery;
- positive correlation was found between healing and perceived social support as well as family social support; social support and recovery were increased together; and
- in addition, negative correlation was found between social support and hopelessness, and hopelessness decreased with the increase of social support level.

Recommendations

NURSES should evaluate the patient with diabetic foot ulcer with all aspects as they do with all other health problems. They should assess the level of hope and social support displayed by patients while they determine the standards of treatment and care. Nurses should implement initiatives to improve outcomes bringing hope to patients. Nurses should carefully assess the social support factors available, and advise the family about how to support the patient. Nurses and other health professionals are also social support factors. Thus, the nurses should be reliable and respond to the calls of patients at all times. Nurses should believe that everyone should be entitled to receive premium personalized holistic treatment, and work for the solution of problems. Both healthcare professionals and patients should be informed about prevention initiatives related to diabetic foot, which have recently become current in our country. Specialized modern diabetic foot clinics should be equipped to coordinate preventive care, AND all diabetes patients should get regular foot examinations.

REFERENCES

[1] IDF. 2013. *Diabetes Atlas 6th edition.* Epub ahead of print 20 April 2011. ISBN: 2-930229-85-3.
[2] RPSGB.2001. *Diabetes Task Force: Practice Guidance for Community Pharmacists on the Care of People with Diabetes.* 2nd ed. London.
[3] Satman, İ., Ömer, B., Tütüncuü, Y., Kalaca, S., Gedik, S., Dinççag, N., Karşıdağ, K., Genç, S. Telci, A., Canbaz, B., Turker, F., Yilmaz, T., Cakir, B., Tuomilehto, J. 2013. "Twelve-year trends in the prevalence and risk factors of diabetes and prediabetes in Turkish adults." *European Journal of Epidemiology.* (TURDEP II GROUP); 28(2):169-180.
[4] Cihangiroğlu M. 2009. "Diabetic Foot Care with Interventional Radiology." *Diabetes Forum* 2009; 5(3):1-7.
[5] Edmonds M. E. 2008. Foster A. V. M, Sanders L. J. *Apractical Manuel of Diabetic foot care*, 2th ed, Blackwell Publishing.
[6] Zeleníková, R., Bužgová, R., Janíková, E., Jarošová, D. 2013. *"Evaluation of Quality of Life of Patients with Diabetic Foot Syndrome in Selected Health Care Facilities of Moravian Silesian Region"* Department of Nursing and Midwifery, Faculty of Medicine, University of Ostrava, Czech Republic.
[7] Boulton, J. M. 2013. "The Diabetic Foot." *Clinics Reviews Articles* (online) Medical Clinics of North America, ISBN: 13:978-1-4557-7598-9 (accessed 1th May 2014) http://www.google.com.tr/books?hl=tr&lr=&id=nenTAAAAQBAJ&oi=fnd&pg=PP1&dq=boulton+2013&ots=pqQqLCAcSy&sig=gX4OIrgPUMjLMuZNqobwQudmLnc&redir_esc=y#v=onepage&q=boulton%202013&f=false.

[8] Jeffcoate W. J., Harding K. G. 2003. "Diabetic foot ulcers." *Lancet*, 361:1545-51.
[9] Reiber G. E., Bowker J. H., Pfefier M. A.2001. *Epidemiology of Foot Ulcers and Amputation in the Diabetic Foot*. 6th ed, p.1332.
[10] National Institute for Health and Clinical Excellence (NICE) 2011. *Diabetic foot problems*. (accessed March 2013) https://www.nice.org.uk/ guidance/ng19/resources/diabetic-foot-problems-prevention-and-management-pdf-1837279828933
[11] Boulton A. J., Vileikyte L., Ragnarson-Tennvall G. 2005. "*The global burden of diabetic foot disease.*" *Lancet*, 366(9498): 1719-1724.
[12] Arslantaş H., Adana F., Kaya F., Turan D. 2010. "*Hopelessness and social support levels in hospitalized patients and the factors affecting them.*" İ. U. F. N. *Journal of Nursing* 2010; 18 (2): 87-97.
[13] Aşti T. Kara M. İpek G. Erci B. 2003."The experiences of loneliness, depression, and social support of Turkish patients with continuous ambulatory peritoneal dialysis and their caregivers." *Journal of Clinical Nursing*, 15 (4): 490–497.
[14] Ginkgos T., Astan G. V. 2006. "Social support, locus of control, and depressive symptoms in hemodialysis patients." *Scandinavian Journal of Psychology*, 47(3): 203– 208.
[15] Stroebe, W., Zech, E., Stroebe, M., Abakoumkın, G. 2005. "Does social support help in bereavement." *Journal of Social and Clinical Psychology*, 24(7): 1030-1050.
[16] Karasar N. 2013. *Research Methodology*, TR, 25th edition.
[17] Hanft J., Surprenant M., Buttita O. 2013. "Wound Managenet, Improving Diabetic Wound Care Outcomes: A Practical Guide." *Podiatry Management* 117-120.
[18] Sheehan P., Jones P., Caselli A., Giurini J. M., Veves A. 2003. "Percent Change in Wound Area of Diabetic Foot Ulcers Over a 4-Week Periods Is a Robust Predictor of Comlete Healing in a 12-Week Prespective Trial." *Diabetes Care* 26(6):1879-1882).
[19] Apelqvist K., Bakker W. H., van Houtum N. C., Schaper. 2008. " Practical guidelines on the management and prevention of the

diabetic foot, Based upon the International Consensus on the Diabetic Foot, Prepared by the International Working Group on the Diabetic Foot." *Diabetes/Metabolism Research and Reviews* 24(1): 181-187.
[20] Delmas L. 2006. "Best practice in the assessment and management of diabetic foot ulcers." *Rehabilitation Nursing, ProQuest Health & Medical Complete* 31 (6): 228.
[21] Royal College of Nursing. 2005. The management of pressure ulcers in primary and secondary care, *A Clinical Practice Guideline* 2005.
[22] Vuorisalo S., Venermo M., LepÃntalo M. 2009. "Treatment of diabetic foot ulcers." *Journal of Cardiovascular Surgery* 50(3): 275.
[23] Çetinkalp Ş. 1998. *Protectiob of Treated Diabetic Foot, Diabetic Foot and treatment*, Ed. M. Tüzün, İzmir, Asya Medical Publishing TR 108-111.
[24] IDF. 2005. *Global Guideline for Type 2 Diabetes*. Chapter 15: Foot Care, 58-62.
[25] RNAO (Registered Nurses Association of Ontorio). 2014. "Assessment and Management of Foot Ulcers for People with Diabetes." *Nursing Best Practice Guidelines Program. Ontorio*, (accessed Ocak 2014) [http://www.rnao.org/Storage/11/536_BPG_Assessment_Foot_Ulcer.pdf.
[26] Thomas-Ramouta, C., Tıerney E., Frykberg R.2010. "Osteomyelitis and lower extremity amputations in the diabetic population." *The Journal of Diabetic Foot Complications* 2010; 2(1):18-27.
[27] Yıldız E. 2012. *Determining the Relationship between Perceived Social Support and Depression Levels in Patient with Diabetic Foot.* Master Thesis, Istanbul University, Institute of Health Sciences, TR,
[28] Hosley J. B., Molle-Mathews E. A. 1999. *Lippincott's textbook for clinical medical assisting*. Wolter Kluwer Company, Philadelphia 320-34.
[29] Bulut I. 2000. *Family Assessment Handbook*, Özel İş Printing, Ankara.
[30] Sorias O. 1992. *Hasta ve sağlıklı öğrencilerde yaşam stresi; sosyal destek ve ruhsal hastalık ilişkisinin incelenmesi* [*Life stress in sick and healthy students; the relationship between social support and*

mental illness]. Seminer Psikoloji Dergisi E. Ü Edebiyat Fakültesi Yayını 33-49.

[31] Uchino N., Uno D, Holt-Lunstad J. 1999. "Social support, physiological processes, and health." *Current Direction in Psychological Science* (5):145- 148.

[32] Karakurt P. R. Hacihasanoğlu Aşilar, Yildirim A. 2013. "Evaluation of the Self-Care Agency and Perceived Social Support in Patients with Diabetes Mellitus." *Journal of Adnan Menderes University Medical Faculty* 14(1): 001-009.

[33] Gallant M. P. 2003. "The influence of social support on chronic illness self-management: A review and directions for research." *Health Education & Behavior* 30(2):170-195.

[34] Choi S. E., Rush E. B., Henry S. L. 2013. "Negative emotions and risk for type 2 diabetes among Korean immigrants." *Diabetes Education.* 39(5):679-688.

[35] Pompili M., Lester D., Innamorati M., De Pisa E., Amore M., Ferrara C., Tatarelli R., Girardi P. 2009. "Quality of life and suicide risk in patients with diabetes mellitus." *Psychosomatics* 50(1):16-23.

[36] Baettie A. M., Campbell R., Vedhara K.2013. "What ever I do it's a lost cause.' The emotional and behavioural experiences of individuals who are ulcer free living with the threat of developing further diabetic foot ulcers: a qualitative interview study." *Health Expectations* 17(3):429-439.

[37] Pedersen S. S., Denollet J., Erdman R. A. M., Serrys P. W., van Domburg R. T. 2009. "Co-occurrence of diabetes and hopelessness predicts adverse prognosis following percutaneous coronary intervention." *Journal of Behavioral Medicine* 32(3): 294-301.

[38] Ceretta L. B., Réus G. Z. 2012. "Abelaira H. M., Jornada L. K., Schwalm M. T., Hoepers N. J., Tomazzi C. D., Gulbis K. G., Ceretta R. A., Quevedo J. Increased prevalence of mood disorders and suicidal ideation in type 2 diabetic patients." *Acta Diabetol* 49(1):227-234.

[39] Jain R., Jain S., Raison C. L., Maletic V. 2011. "Painful diabetic neuropathy is more than pain alone: examining the role of anxiety

and depression as mediators and complicators." *Current Diabetes Reports* 11(4): 275-284.
[40] Salomé G. M., Alves S. G., Costa V. F., Pereira V. R., Ferreira L. M. 2013. "Feelings of powerlessness and hope for cure in patients with chronic lower-limb ulcers." *Journal of Wound Care* 22(6):300 – 304.
[41] Alexander S. J. 2013. "Time to get serious about assessing – and managing – psychosocial issues associated with chronic wounds." *Curr Opin Support Palliat Care* 7(1).95-100.
[42] Jensen B. O., Petersson K. 2003. "The illness experiences of patients after a first time myocardial infarction." *Patient Education and Counseling* 51(2):123-31.
[43] Abramson I., Metalsky G. L., Alloy L. B. 1989. "Hopelessness depression: A theory-based subtype of depression." *Psychological Review,* 96(2):358-372.
[44] Tan M., Karabulutlu E., Okanlı A., Erdem N. 2005. "The Evaluation of Relationship between Social Support and Hopelessness in Hemodialysis Patients." *Journal of Ataturk University Nursing School* 8 (2):32-39.
[45] Holder B. 1997. "Family support and survival among African-America end-stage renal disease patients." *Adv Ren Replace Ther* 4(1):13-21.
[46] Soykan A., Arapaslan B., Kumbasar H. 2003. "Suicidal behavior, satisfaction with life, and perceived social support in end-stage renal disease." *Transplantation Proceedings* 35(4):1290-1291.
[47] Christensen A. J., Smith T. W., Turner C. W. 1992. "Family support, physical impairment, and adherence in hemodialysis: an investigation of main and buffering effects." *Journal of Behavioral Medicine* 15(4):313-325.
[48] Christensen A. J., Wiebe J. S., Smith T. W. 1994. "Predictors of survival among hemodialysis patients: effect of perceived family support." *Health Psychol* 13(6):521-5.

INDEX

A

Advanced Glycocylated End Products (AGEs), 23
advanced therapies, 82, 86, 87, 114, 116
allografts, 27, 94
amniotic fluid, 31, 44
AMP, x, 52, 56, 57, 58, 59, 60, 61, 62, 63, 64, 65, 66
angiogenesis, ix, 20, 28, 36, 38, 42, 43, 45, 49, 58, 92, 93, 94, 96, 98, 100, 101, 102, 127, 133, 141, 145
antibiotic, vii, ix, x, 52, 54, 56, 61, 63, 67, 70, 72, 73, 74, 77, 85, 88, 109, 110, 121
antibiotic resistance, ix, 52, 56, 61, 70, 72, 73, 77, 85, 109
antibiotic resistant, vii, x, 52, 54, 56, 61, 63, 67, 74, 88, 110, 121
antimicrobial peptides, v, vii, x, 51, 52, 56, 58, 60, 61, 68, 69, 70, 71, 72, 73, 74, 75, 76, 77, 78, 79
antiseptics, xi, 82, 86, 87, 88, 89, 90, 92, 114, 128, 129, 134
autografts, 27

B

bacteriophage, xi, 82, 86, 108, 109, 110, 111, 112, 113, 116, 125, 147
bacteriophage therapy, xi, 82, 86, 108, 109, 110, 111, 112, 113, 116, 125, 147
bio-engineered skin, xi, 82, 86, 87, 90, 114
biofilm, ix, 26, 52, 53, 54, 55, 56, 59, 61, 63, 65, 67, 68, 69, 70, 71, 72, 73, 75, 76, 77, 84, 85, 88, 90, 112, 116, 122, 129, 130, 133, 135
bone, 20, 31, 33, 34, 38, 41, 42, 43, 44, 46, 49, 104
bone XE "bone" marrow, 20, 31, 33, 34, 38, 41, 42, 43, 44, 46, 49, 104

C

cardiovascular disease, 23
chronic wound, 27, 29, 37, 40, 42, 56, 73, 83, 88, 89, 98, 99, 112, 123, 127, 128, 136, 140, 142, 143, 145, 169
cold / hot stress, 2
collagen, 27, 28, 29, 34, 38, 58, 91, 93, 95, 99, 101, 115
cytokine, 37, 38, 58, 100, 104, 120

D

depression, 25, 161, 166, 167, 169
diabetes, v, vii, viii, ix, x, xi, 1, 2, 3, 4, 5, 7, 8, 15, 16, 17, 19, 20, 21, 22, 23, 24, 25, 26, 42, 43, 47, 48, 49, 51, 53, 54, 55, 65, 67, 68, 69, 75, 77, 78, 81, 82, 83, 84, 100, 104, 118, 119, 120, 121, 123, 124, 126, 128, 129, 130, 131, 132, 134, 136, 139,140, 141, 145, 146, 147, 148, 152, 154, 155, 156, 157, 159, 160, 161, 163, 165, 166, 167, 168, 169
diabetes foot ulcer, ix, 20
diabetes mellitus, viii, 5, 17, 19, 20, 21, 22, 43, 49, 55, 65, 121, 123, 152, 160, 161, 168
diabetic foot infection (DFI), v, vii, ix, 52, 53, 54, 55, 56, 61, 63, 64, 65, 66, 67, 70, 73, 74, 75, 83, 84, 85, 86, 88, 104, 112, 116, 121, 122, 124, 126, 132, 134, 135, 145
diabetic foot ulcers, v, vi, vii, x, xi, 19, 26, 43, 46, 63, 68, 70, 72, 76, 77, 81, 82, 83, 87, 118, 119, 120, 122, 124, 125, 128, 129, 130, 131, 132, 133, 134, 136, 137, 138, 139, 140, 144, 146, 147, 148, 151, 152, 154, 155, 160, 163, 164, 166, 167, 168
differentiation, vii, ix, 20, 31, 33, 34, 38, 39, 45, 49, 58, 104

E

electrical stimulation, xi, 82, 86, 97, 120, 125, 140, 141, 143, 145, 147
embryonic stem (ES), 30, 97, 98, 99, 115

F

fibroblasts, 27, 28, 29, 31, 32, 35, 38, 48, 58, 88, 91, 93, 100, 101, 102, 107, 142, 147
foot ulcer, vii, viii, ix, xi, 1, 7, 19, 20, 24, 25, 26, 36, 51, 53, 68, 78, 83, 84, 86, 92, 100, 101, 114, 121, 123, 124, 125, 126, 127, 129, 130, 131, 133, 134, 135, 136, 145, 146, 147, 148, 151, 152, 153, 155, 156, 160, 161, 163, 164, 166, 167

G

glycosaminoglycans, 28, 93
granulocyte-colony stimulating factor, xi, 82, 86, 104, 126, 141, 142
growth, xi, 82, 86, 99, 115, 133, 144, 147

H

hematopoietic stem cells (HSCs), 30, 35
hope, vi, xi, 132, 151, 153, 160, 161, 162, 163, 164, 169
human, xi, 82, 86, 99, 115, 133, 144, 147
hyperbaric oxygen therapy, xi, 82, 86, 102, 117, 121, 123, 124, 138, 140, 145, 148
hyperglycemia, 23, 25, 83, 100, 134, 155

I

induced pluripotent stem (iPS), 30
insulin, 3, 4, 20, 21, 22, 38, 82, 121, 156, 157

K

keratinocytes, 27, 28, 29, 38, 39, 58, 88, 91, 99, 147

Index

L

light, xi, 82, 86, 106, 131, 145
low-level light therapy, xi, 82, 86, 106, 131, 145

M

machine vision, v, 1, 2, 16
macrophages, 28, 37, 47, 58, 91, 98, 99, 100, 102, 105
mesenchymal stem cells, v, ix, 19, 20, 30, 31, 32, 44, 45, 49
microcirculation, 35, 36, 107

N

negative pressure wound therapy, xi, 82, 86, 95, 118, 120, 128, 136, 137, 148
nephropathy, 24
neuropathy, viii, ix, 1, 2, 6, 7, 8, 10, 11, 15, 16, 17, 18, 23, 26, 51, 53, 83, 84, 156, 161, 163, 168
nisin, x, 52, 57, 61, 62, 63, 66, 67, 68, 69, 71, 73, 74, 78

O

off-loading, 41, 118, 163

P

P. aeruginosa, 54, 64, 66, 89, 90, 112, 113
paracrine, ix, 20, 35, 38, 43
pexiganan, x, 52, 61, 63, 64, 66, 70, 71, 72
pro-inflammatory, 37, 96
pseudomonas aeruginosa, 54, 70, 73, 88, 129, 130

R

recombinant human platelet-derived growth factor, xi, 82, 86, 99, 115, 133, 144, 147
retinopathy, viii, 1, 24

S

S. aureus, 54, 55, 63, 64, 66, 84, 89, 90, 110, 112, 113
social support, vi, vii, xi, 151, 152, 153, 154, 157, 158, 159, 160, 161, 162, 163, 164, 166, 167, 168, 169
staphylococcus aureus, 54, 69, 71, 73, 75, 76, 77, 83, 124, 129, 135

T

Type 1 diabetes, 3, 4, 21
Type 2 diabetes, 3, 4, 17, 18, 21, 167

W

wound healing, ix, x, xi, 20, 27, 28, 29, 30, 34, 36, 37, 38, 39, 41, 42, 43, 44, 45, 46, 49, 52, 54, 56, 58, 75, 81, 85, 86, 92, 96, 97, 98, 99, 100, 101, 103, 104, 105, 115, 116, 120, 123, 124, 125, 126, 127, 128, 129, 130, 131, 133, 134, 139, 141, 142, 144, 145, 146, 147, 148, 149, 152, 154, 155, 159, 161, 162

Related Nova Publications

CYSTIC TUMORS OF THE PANCREAS

EDITOR: Robert Grützmann, M.D., Ph.D.

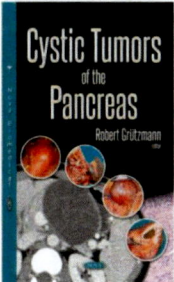

SERIES: Endocrinology Research and Clinical Developments

BOOK DESCRIPTION: Cystic tumors of the pancreas today are diagnosed more frequently in clinical practice, mainly due to an increased use of the modern advanced imaging modalities. Bland cysts of the pancreas most often develop after chronic or acute inflammation of the pancreas. However, the current knowledge concerning the development of cystic neoplasias of the pancreas is still rudimentary.

HARDCOVER ISBN: 978-1-53612-523-8
RETAIL PRICE: $160

PINEAL GLAND: RESEARCH ADVANCES AND CLINICAL CHALLENGES

EDITOR: Angel Catalá, Ph.D.

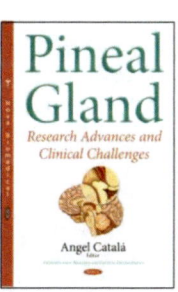

SERIES: Endocrinology Research and Clinical Developments

BOOK DESCRIPTION: This book presents an overview of the research advances and clinical challenges of the pineal gland. The topics analyzed cover a broad spectrum of functions played by the pineal gland and present new information in this area of research.

HARDCOVER ISBN: 978-1-53612-117-9
RETAIL PRICE: $230

To see a complete list of Nova publications, please visit our website at www.novapublishers.com

Related Nova Publications

USES OF ELECTRICAL STIMULATION FOR DIGESTIVE AND ENDOCRINE SURGEONS

EDITOR: Jaime Ruiz-Tovar, M.D., Ph.D.

SERIES: Endocrinology Research and Clinical Developments

BOOK DESCRIPTION: The use of electrical stimulators with medical aims has increased exponentially in the last years. The uses are very different. Though the most widely known are referred to as the approaches performed by neurosurgeons, evidence has recently appeared, supporting its use by many other medical specialties.

SOFTCOVER ISBN: 978-1-53615-036-0
RETAIL PRICE: $95

SEROTONIN AND DOPAMINE RECEPTORS: FUNCTIONS, SYNTHESIS AND HEALTH EFFECTS

EDITORS: Monica Munoz and Marshall Mckinney

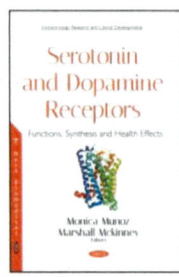

SERIES: Endocrinology Research and Clinical Developments

BOOK DESCRIPTION: In this compilation, the authors begin with a review of the mechanisms of synthesis and secretion, cellular effects and the involvement of serotonin (5-HT) in physiological and behavioral functions horses.

SOFTCOVER ISBN: 978-1-53613-216-8
RETAIL PRICE: $95

To see a complete list of Nova publications, please visit our website at www.novapublishers.com